Iron Metabolism in Infants

Editor
Bo Lönnerdal, Ph.D.
Professor
Department of Nutrition
University of California
Davis, California

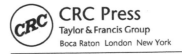

CRC Press
Taylor & Francis Group
Boca Raton London New York

CRC Press is an imprint of the
Taylor & Francis Group, an **informa** business

CRC Press
Taylor & Francis Group
6000 Broken Sound Parkway NW, Suite 300
Boca Raton, FL 33487-2742

ISBN 13: 978-0-367-45089-2 (pbk)
ISBN 13: 978-0-8493-5433-5 (hbk)

Visit the Taylor & Francis Web site at
http://www.taylorandfrancis.com

and the CRC Press Web site at
http://www.crcpress.com

Library of Congress Cataloging-in-Publication Data

Iron metabolism in infants / editor, Bo Lonnerdal.
   p.   cm.
   Includes bibliographies and index.
   ISBN 0-8493-5433-1
   1. Infants—Metabolism. 2 Iron—Metabolism. 3. Infants—Nutrition. 4. Baby food—Iron content. 5. Iron deficiency diseases in infants—Pathogenesis.
I. Lonnerdal, Bo, 1938-
[DNLM: 1. Anemia, Hypochromic—in infancy & childhood. 2. Anemia, Hypochromic—prevention & control. 3. Food, Fortified. 4. Iron—metabolism. WH 160 I713]
RJ128.I76 1990   618.92'396—dc20   89-10023 CIP
DNLM/DLC for Library of Congress

Library of Congress Card Number 89-10023

PREFACE

Iron deficiency is prevalent among infants and children in many parts of the world. As long-term iron deficiency anemia has been correlated to impaired immune competence, higher incidence of infection, learning disabilities, and physical inactivity, prevention of iron deficiency is a primary objective for pediatricians, nutritionists, and health care professionals around the world. It, therefore, becomes important to obtain further knowledge about the causes of iron deficiency, its manifestations, and its prevention.

The purpose of this book is to integrate several aspects of iron metabolism in infants and to present the forefront of the research in different topic areas. While performing this task I have had the privilege of working with the most knowledgeable researchers available in this field and I am grateful for their contributions. Dr. Helmut Huebers has written two chapters on iron metabolism and the function of iron-binding proteins. These chapters are up-to-date reviews, presenting and discussing recently obtained information on mechanisms of iron absorption, transport, and storage. Dr. Martti Siimes describes the particular problems of premature infants as they relate to iron accumulation, hemoglobin synthesis, and overall iron status. The potential toxic effects of iron, particularly through the formation of free radicals and, in turn, its consequences for lipid peroxidation and membrane integrity are described by Dr. Lennart Jansson. In my chapter, I have attempted to present our state of knowledge regarding the bioavailability of iron from various food sources, such as human milk, cow's milk formula and soy formula. Drs. Sean Lynch and Richard Hurrell present the practical considerations and their implications for iron fortification of infant formulas. In the last chapter, Dr. Tomás Walter and colleagues describe their successful field trials of various ways of fortifying formulas and foods for infants and children. This chapter appropriately demonstrates how all the information presented in the previous chapters can be used in an attempt to minimize the risk of iron deficiency.

Finally, we would all like to dedicate this book to the memory of Dr. Abraham Stekel. Abe, who was a highly appreciated colleague and friend to all of us, had accepted the invitation to write a chapter for this book — unfortunately his untimely death made this impossible and the task was completed by members of his research group at INTA. We all miss him deeply.

Bo Lönnerdal, Ph.D.

THE EDITOR

Bo Lönnerdal, Ph.D., is Professor of Nutrition in the College of Agricultural and Environmental Sciences at the University of California at Davis. He also has a joint appointment as Professor of Internal Medicine, School of Medicine at UC Davis.

Dr. Lönnerdal obtained his training at the University of Uppsala, Sweden, receiving his B.Sc. in 1969. He obtained his M.S. and Ph.D. degrees in 1972 and 1973, respectively, from the Department of Biochemistry, University of Uppsala. After doing postdoctoral work at the Institute of Nutrition, University of Uppsala, he was appointed Assistant Professor of Nutrition at the same university in 1976. In 1978 Dr. Lönnerdal received a Fellowship to go the Department of Nutrition at the University of California, Davis. After a period as Visiting Research Nutritionist, Dr. Lönnerdal was appointed Assistant Professor in 1981, Associate Professor in 1983, and Professor in 1985. He was also appointed Professor of Internal Medicine in 1986.

Dr. Lönnerdal is a member of the American Institute of Nutrition, American Society for Clinical Nutrition, Society for Experimental Biology and Medicine, and the Swedish Nutrition Society.

He has been the recipient of the Henning Throne-Holst Fellowship in Nutrition & Physiology (1978-79); St. Göran's Lectureship in Pediatrics at Karolinska Institute, Stockholm, Sweden and University of Copenhagen, Denmark (1986); and given the Eric Underwood Memorial Lecture at the Sixth International Conference on Trace Elements in Man and Animals (TEMA-6) in 1987. He was also Visiting Professor at the Department of Pediatrics, McMaster University, Hamilton, Ontario, Canada (1987).

Dr. Lönnerdal has been the recipient of research grants from the National Institutes of Health, the U.S. Department of Agriculture Competitive Grants Program, Wisconsin Milk Marketing Board, and private industry. He has published more than 200 papers. His current research interests are in pediatric nutrition and trace element metabolism.

CONTRIBUTORS

Eva Hertrampf, M.D.
Assistant Professor
Hematology Unit
University of Chile Institute of Nutrition
  and Food Technology
Santiago, Chile

Helmut A. Huebers, Ph.D.
Department of Pediatrics
Baylor College of Medicine
Texas Medical Center
Houston, Texas

Richard F. Hurrell, Ph.D.
Department of Research
Nestlé Products
La Tour de Peilz, Switzerland

Lennart T. Jansson, M.D.
Assistant Professor
Department of Pediatrics
Central Hospital
Kristianstad, Sweden

Bo Lönnerdal, Ph.D.
Professor
Department of Nutrition
University of California
Davis, California

Sean R. Lynch, M.D.
Department of Medicine
University of Kansas Medical Center
Kansas City, Kansas

Manuel Olivares, M.D.
Assistant Professor
Hematology Unit
University of Chile Institute of Nutrition
  and Food Technology
Santiago, Chile

Martti A. Siimes, M.D.
Assistant Professor
Pediatric Hematology Division
University of Helsinki
Helsinki, Finland

Tomás Walter, M.D.
Professor and Head
Associate Department of Hematology
University of Chile Institute of Nutrition
  and Food Technology
Santiago, Chile

TABLE OF CONTENTS

Chapter 1

IRON METABOLISM: IRON TRANSPORT AND CELLULAR UPTAKE MECHANISMS

Helmut A. Huebers

TABLE OF CONTENTS

I. INTRODUCTION

It is unlikely that life on earth could have evolved without iron.[1-4] There are many good reasons for this conclusion. First of all, the presence of enormous quantities of this metal in the earth's core resulted and still results in the formation of an effective magnetic shield deflecting various forms of noxious solar and cosmic radiation. Secondly, on the crust of the earth, iron is unsurpassed in its versatility as a catalyst for basic metabolic processes, and most importantly, at the time life began, iron was readily available in a relatively nontoxic form to act as a catalyst for the life processes which evolved.

Iron is a reactive metal and so is rarely found free in nature, except in meteorites. It has ready access to the ferrous and ferric oxidation state which permits catalysis in a whole array of important biochemical reactions in the form of heme and nonheme enzymes. These include electron transfer, the transport, storage, and activation of oxygen, nitrogen fixation, detoxification of activated oxygen species, and deoxyribonucleotide synthesis from ribonucleoside diphosphates.[5,6] The chemical properties of iron which allow this versatility also lead to the paradoxical situation that the fourth most abundant metal in the biosphere is exceedingly difficult to assimilate. Procurement of iron from external sources presented no problem in the early days of the planet and soluble ferrous iron was abundant in the reductive atmosphere present then. With the evolution of the blue-green algae and photosynthesis, however, oxygen appeared in the atmosphere leading to the ability of the iron to oxidize to the ferric form which is far more insoluble than the ferrous form. Thus, the precipitation of large amounts of iron from the waters of the earth reduce the availability of iron to living organisms. As a consequence, the organisms evolved mechanisms specifically adapted to the acquisition of iron. In the microorganisms, this is expressed in the development of siderophores, a very large variety of iron chelating substances which can chelate the iron in the environment and make it available to the organism.[7] In higher forms and in man, a multifaceted absorptive and distribution system has developed, involving solubilization of iron by gastric acid, its protein-mediated absorption in the mucosal cells of the upper duodenum, and protein-mediated distribution within the body.[8-11]

During the processes of absorption and distribution, iron is almost always tightly bound to proteins, leaving an extremely low concentration of "free iron". This is important because relatively low concentrations of free intracellular iron result in severe damage to a number of cellular constituents including membranes and DNA.[2,12-15] All these properties make it very clear that for life to continue in the presence of iron and oxygen, specific carriers had to be evolved. They must function not only to keep iron in soluble and bioavailable form, but to keep it in a benign state where it does not catalyze toxic side reactions and which enable iron to cross cell membranes in an innocent way.[4,9,16]

While a variety of transport mechanisms are seen in invertebrates,[17,18] vertebrate species have consistently utilized a special transport protein of about 80,000 mol wt which possesses two high affinity biding sites for iron. This glycoprotein was first isolated and characterized by Schade and Caroline.[19] Laurell and Ingelman called it transferrin because of its iron transport function.[20] Since then, the chemistry and functional importance of the transferrin class of proteins including the lactoferrins has been well documented.[4,9,10,21-29]

Although transferrin can transport and procure iron, a second device was needed to permit its appropriate delivery to body tissues. Hidden from the investigative eye until the last few years was a membrane receptor system specific for transferrin.[30-34] These receptors bind the transferrin iron complex at the cell surface and permit iron transport into the cell.

An understanding of the behavior of the transferrin molecule and its tissue receptor is necessary if one wishes to study the pathways of body iron exchange. We will take a look at the working of these components of iron metabolism, how they are regulated, and how this knowledge may be used to evaluate the iron status of individuals. Special attention will

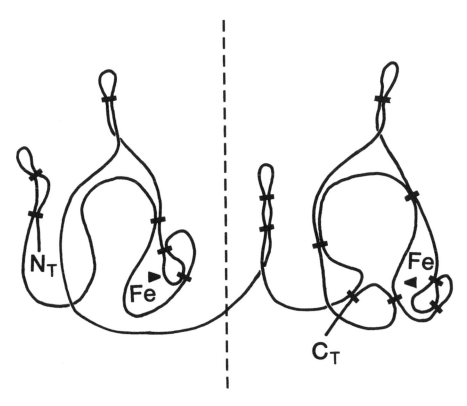

FIGURE 1.   A string model of the polypeptide chain of transferrin including the internal disulfide bridges. There are two large independent and similar, but not identical, globular domains, each of which can bind one ferric iron. The N terminal half is on the left. The figure is adapted from ovotransferrin as shown in References 24 and 26.

be given to the discussion of features pertinent to the physiology and pathophysiology of the iron metabolism in infants.

II. TRANSFERRIN

Transferrins, so-called because of their iron transport function, are a class of related metal binding glycoproteins with specificity for ferric iron.[4,20,21] Serum transferrin from many vertebrate species, especially the higher mammals, has been thoroughly characterized. Each transferrin is a single polypeptide chain glycoprotein with molecular weight estimates between 75,000 and 85,000.[10,24,35,36] In humans, serum transferrin consists of a single polypeptide chain of 678 amino acid residues which together with the two oligosaccharide chains gives a calculated molecular weight of 79,570.[37,38] Transferrin has a three-dimensional globular, bilobal structure.[39,40] The two lobes may correspond to N- and C-terminal domains of the molecule (Figure 1). Ever since it was appreciated that this single polypeptide chain had two metal binding sites buried in the N- and C-terminal portions of the molecule, there has been speculation that transferrin evolved as a result of gene duplication and fusion. As a matter of fact, there is a high degree of internal homology between the two halves of the transferrin molecule.[23,29,41-44] These homologous domains which comprise amino acid residue 1 through 336 and 337 to 679, respectively, give about 40% identical residues, possibly reflecting functional constraints associated with iron binding or binding to its receptor.[42,45] Williams[26] has suggested the importance of disulfide groups in stabilizing the iron binding site in trying to trace the evolution of the development of the 17 disulfides found in human transferrin (Figure 1).

Utilization of newer techniques to isolate transferrin cDNA has further underlined this homology. When cDNA sequences of the N and C domains where compared by statistical analysis, three regions of extensive internal nucleotides sequence homology were identified.[38,46] These regions demonstrated 72, 64, and 62% homology, respectively, as compared to the 40% homology obtained when the entire N and C domains are compared.[42,45] Intensive search for single-sided transferrin molecules has led to the discovery of such an iron-binding protein of about 40,000 Da in the invertebrate *Pyura stolonifera*.[17] One reason for the duplication of the molecule in invertebrates was probably the development of a secretory kidney which would have excreted the molecule of 40,000 Da.[18,26]

While iron is complexed by transferrin in ferric form, ferrous iron added to plasma binds more completely, presumably because ferric iron is rapidly hydrolyzed to unreactive forms while ferrous iron is bound to transferrin before much hydrolysis occurs. Analysis of human transferrins by spectroscopy and chemical modification reveals that the binding sites for Fe^{3+} are probably located near the junction of the two peptide fragments joined by disulfide bridge 3 (CYS 117 to CYS 194) and in the N-terminal domain.[47] The two iron molecules have been estimated to be 25 to 43 Å apart.[48,49] TRY 185 to TRY 188 and two of the three histidines, probably serve as ligands to the metal.[47] The ligands which can bind the iron are contributed partly by the protein and partly by an anion, usually bicarbonate or carbonate.[50,51] This is one of the most characteristic properties of iron binding by transferrin.[4,10,24,51] The function of the anion is to lock the iron into place in the molecule by serving as a bridging ligand between iron and protein, thus making a coordination site on the iron unavailable to water. It is likely that ARG 124 (and/or the cluster LYS 115, LYS 116, His-119) is at the carbonate binding site which would enable the anion to coordinate the iron as well.[47] In the absence of the anion, the affinity of transferrin for iron is virtually zero. The carbonate also appears crucial in iron release.[52,53] Since this anion bound to transferrin is too strong as to preclude a simple dissociation mechanism for the release of iron, it may well be that the primary event *in vivo* is a protonal attack on the anion, following which disruption of the metal protein bond readily occurs. That such a mechanism is necessary is underlined by the fact that under physiological conditions, the apparent stability constants for the two iron binding sites on transferrin are in the range of 10^{19} to 10^{20} M^{-1}.[10,21,54]

In the absence of iron, the binding sites of transferrin can accommodate other metals including gallium, copper, chromium, cobalt, manganese, vanadium, aluminum, terbium, plutonium, europium, indium, and platinum.[49,55-63] It is also possible that transferrin functions *in vivo* as a transport agent for Cr^{3+}, Mn^{3+}, and Zn^{2+} as well as for plutonium, americum, and curium.[55,64-66] Gallium bound by transferrin has also been considered useful in transporting this metal to receptor-rich tissues.[67-70] Demonstration of *in vitro* binding, however, should not be taken as adequate evidence. For example, copper binds to apotransferrin *in vitro*.[71] There is no copper demonstrable in transferrin precipitated from normal plasma by transferrin antibody despite the presence of open binding sites and the amount of copper equivalent to plasma iron.[297]

The two metal binding sites of transferrin are similar but not identical based on physical measurements. Perhaps the most interesting difference, which may have functional implications, is the finding that in the human transferrin the N terminal binding site is relatively acid labile in that iron is released at a higher pH than iron bound to the binding site of the C-terminal domain.[72-74]

All the transferrins examined so far are glycoproteins and there are marked variations in the number and composition of the carbohydrate group, the amount in different species varying from 2 to 12%.[75] The carbohydrate moiety of human transferrins was reported to contain biantennary, triantennary, and quarterantennary glycans with different number of sialic acid residues.[43,76,77] The carbohydrate contents of transferrins isolated from different tissues in one species may be quite different; e.g., in the hen, the protein moieties of serum transferrin and ovotransferrin appear to be identical, but the carbohydrate groups are different.[21] The two glycans of human transferrin which contain 6% carbohydrate by weight have been extensively studied.[43,77] The sequence of each chain appears to be identical with each made up of two branches so as to be characterized as biantennary. Further work has indicated that the chains are joined by β-N-glycosidic linkages to the asparagine residue 415 and 608, both of which are in the C-terminal domain of the protein. Differences in glycan site and side chains account largely for differences in chemical behavior between plasma transferrin, ovotransferrin, testicular transferrin, and central nervous system transferrin.[21,43,77-80]

The function and significance of the carbohydrate residues found on transferrin are presently unknown. The interaction of transferrin with receptors appears to be unaffected by neuraminidase treatment.[81,82] A deviation from the biantennary structure, for example, may explain why different preparations of desialated transferrin have a diffferential uptake by the asialoglycoprotein receptor which is present on hepatocytes and may provide the mechanism for the initiation of catabolic breakdown of serum transferrin.[83-85] Of additional interest is the observation that while some desialation of transferrin does occur, this is not irreversible.[86,87] The altered transferrin can be resialated within the hepatocyte and returned to the plasma. Impairment in this function may account for the increase in desialated transferrin seen in the alcoholic.[88,89]

The physical structure of purified transferrin is similar in crystalline states and in solution. By X-ray analysis, its structure is nearly ellipsoidal.[90] Dielectric dispersion and viscosity measurements of human diferric plasma transferrin solution indicate a prolate ellipsoid shape 11.0×5.5 nm.[39] The ratio of major and minor axis of the apoprotein, considered as an ellipsoid of revolution, is about 3 to 1, decreasing to 2.5 to 1 when iron is bound.[9] The molecular volume of transferrin is determined by the technique of small angle neutron scattering to 144 ± 10^2 Å.[91] X-ray analysis of rabbit serum transferrin indicates a bilobal structure, each lobe of which contains an iron-binding site.[39,40] Saturation of human transferrin with iron alters the conformation sufficient to produce detectable changes in the hydrodynamic properties.[35,92] These studies also indicate that the shape changes are progressive as first and second atoms of iron are added. The binding of iron also alters the position of the N glycans relative to the polypeptide.[85] Binding of metal ions also appears to stabilize the structure of transferrin which is somewhat more compact for the iron-saturated molecule as compared to the apoprotein. The compactness of the metal-loaded protein may explain why it is more resistant to thermal and protolytic attack or to exchange of deuterium with salt and water than the apoprotein.[21,27,92-95]

A. GENETICS

Chromosomal mapping by *in situ* hybridization and somatic cell hybrid analysis indicates that the transferrin gene is located at q21-25 on human chromosome 3, consistent with a linkage between transferrin, transferrin-receptor, and melanoma p97 loci[46,96-99] (Figure 2). An additional study employing genetic linkage analysis of a pedigree heterogeneous for pseudocholinesterase further supported the notion that the transferrin locus is on human chromosome 3.[100] Messenger RNA produced by this gene is about 2400 to 2500 bases long, with a relatively short 3' noncoding sequence of 166 nucleotides and 2037 bases coded for 678 amino acid residues.[37]

Genetic polymorphism of plasma transferrin has been reported in a number of species including man.[25,89,101-103] While some of these relate to changes in carbohydrate side chains,[104] others are due to amino acid substitutions. About 20 human variants of the latter are known, but only 4 of them with a frequency of greater than 1% in the population.[25,105] Three genetic variants of human transferrins: D1, DCHL, and D2, have been characterized and found to differ in single amino acids (ASP to GLY), (HIS to ARG), and (GLY to GLU).[46] The first

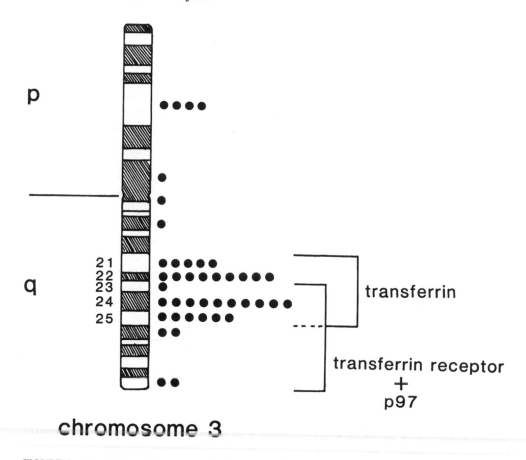

FIGURE 2. Localization of human transferrin gene on chromosome 3 adapted from References 46 and 98; distribution of labeled sites from 60 cells (75% of grains localized to 3q 21-25). Estimates for the localization of the transferrin receptor[96,97,99] and the p97 antigen[293,294] are indicated for comparison.

two have been explained by nucleotide sequence to be mutational transitions (A to G, G to A), respectively, in the second nucleotide of each of the three codons. These variants show no apparent difference in their ability to bind and transport iron.[106] One unusual human transferrin which does bind abnormally has been identified by polyacrylamide gel electrophoresis (PAGE). The variant transferrin, while able to bind two atoms of iron, has a spectral abnormality in the C2 terminal binding site and its iron is dissociated from the protein on electrophoresis in the presence of 6 *M* urea.[107] The iron-free C-terminal domain of the variant protein is less stable than normal to thermal denaturation.

B. PRODUCTION, DISTRIBUTION, AND METABOLISM OF TRANSFERRIN

Although a number of different cells cultured *in situ* have shown the ability to synthesize transferrin, it is generally agreed that almost all serum transferrin is synthesized by the liver.[22] This has been shown most dramatically in a patient undergoing liver transplant, by the plasma isotransferrin profile changed from that of the patient before operation to that of the donor liver.[108] Further documentation includes the finding of large amounts of messenger RNA for transferrin in the chick liver[109,110] and the synthesis with a labeled transferrin from amino acids in liver perfusion studies.[111] Ultrastructural studies of 48-h cultured rat hepatocytes show transferrin located in the endoplasmic reticulum and Golgi apparatus.[112] This intracellular pool can be depleted when transferrin synthesis is stimulated by bleeding.[113]

Hepatic production of transferrin occurs primarily in the hepatocytes as shown in studies of isolated hepatocytes using immunologic techniques,[114,115] and by the presence of specific messenger RNA in chick hepatocytes. The messenger RNA for transferrin is increased with iron deficiency.[109] The protein initially formed is some 19 to 20 amino acids longer than the final molecule, but is later split by proteolysis.[78,116] The molecule also undergoes glycosylation before entering circulation. Inhibition of proteolysis prevents secretion, but inhibition of glycosylation has little effect.[116] The overall rate of transferrin synthesis is about one fifth as great as albumin synthesis.[117]

The other major site of transferrin production is in the lactating mammary gland, where it has been estimated that production exceeds that of the liver.[118,119] Evidence for transferrin synthesis by the central nervous system *in vivo* is also convincing.[79,120] In addition, transferrin synthesis has been demonstrated in Sertoli cells, in lymph nodes, in lymphocytes, in macrophages, in fibroblasts, and in a number of other tissues *in vitro*.[121-126] It seems unlikely that the production of transferrin by these other body cells *in vitro* is of any quantitative importance to the production of plasma transferrin.

As in the case of many other proteins, little information is available on the precise site of mechanism of transferrin catabolism under normal conditions. Studies of isolated perfused liver suggest that this organ may account for 10% of the breakdown. In distinction to many other proteins, desialation has little effect on the rate of catabolism of transferrin.[83,127]

III. TRANSFERRIN RECEPTORS

Experiments performed more than 2 decades ago proved that transferrin bound iron was avidly taken up by reticulocytes.[128] Therefore, the presence of membrane receptors for transferrin of the reticulocytes was postulated, but nearly 20 years elapsed before some understanding of the chemical nature of the receptor was reached.[34,129-134] Early efforts to isolate the receptor by the use of nonionic or ionic detergents initially give conflicting results.[135-137] The situation has become clarified, largely through use of monoclonal antibodies directed against a major human cell surface glycoprotein on proliferating cells.[138] The resulting immunoprecipitate was shown to contain the transferrin receptor.[138-140] Identification of the chemical characteristics of this material served as a standard for the more conventional isolation procedures.

Binding studies used to measure these transferrin receptors were initially performed on hemoglobin-producing cells.[128,133,141-144] They demonstrated that the transferrin receptor expression was related to the rate of hemoglobin production, and thus showed the receptor density was directly related to the cells' iron requirements.[142,145] Transferrin receptors have also been measured on placenta, another tissue with a high iron uptake, since large amounts of iron must be transferred to the fetus, particularly in the later stages of pregnancy. Placenta has not only proved useful in measurements of transferrin binding to isolated cell membrane preparations, but the availability of large amounts of this tissue has permitted the isolation and purification of human transferrin receptor.[34,129,146]

A. STRUCTURE OF THE TRANSFERRIN RECEPTOR

The transferrin receptor is a disulfide-linked transmembrane glycoprotein with a molecular weight of about 180,000,[137,146-148] each receptor binding two molecules of transferrin.[32,149] Treatment with reducing agents leads to cleavage of the single disulfide bridge and formation to two monomers, each 90,000 (Figure 3). Like other receptor proteins, the transferrin receptor is amphipathic, i.e., has two hydrophilic regions which extend into the aqueous medium outside the cell and into the cytoplasm, and a central hydrophobic region that helps to anchor the receptor into the membrane.[32,33,148,150] The hydrophilic cytoplasmic "tail" of the receptor has a molecular weight of about 5000 and frequently contains phosphate bound to the hydroxyl group of a serine residue. The hydrophilic part extending from the

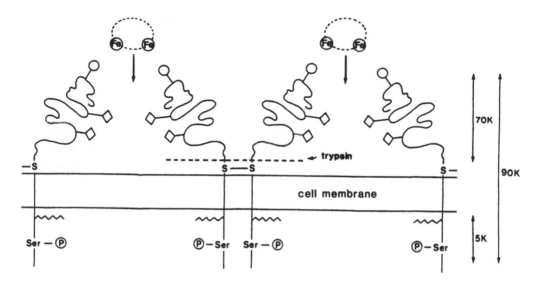

FIGURE 3.   Transferrin receptor. A schematic representation of the cell surface and transferrin receptor. This transmembrane protein consists of two disulfide-bridged monomers with covalently bound fatty acid and complex carbohydrate chains. The receptor model is taken from Reference 32 with changes made to suggest cross-linking of the transferrin receptors after binding transferrin. This could account for the patching or capping phenomenon observed.

surface has a molecular weight of about 140,000. Treatment with trypsin results in the formation of two fragments of 70,000 mol wt each, suggesting cleavage exclusive of the single disulfide bridge. These fragments are still able to bind transferrin. The hydrophobic part of the receptor contains fatty acid residues and palmitate as a result of posttranslational modification.[150,151] Each subunit of the transferrin receptor carries a high mannose and a complex type of oligosaccharide in an *N*-asparagine linkage. The significance of the carbohydrate moiety and of the covalently bound lipid is unknown,[32,150] but an oligosaccharide chain has been claimed to be essential for transferrin binding to reticulocytes.[144]

Each receptor binds two molecules of transferrin, presumably one molecule per polypeptide chain. The transferrin receptors have a very high affinity for diferric transferrin with an estimated association constant in the range of 2 to $7 \times 10^{-9} M$.[32,33,148] This allows the iron-loaded transferrin to be bound by its receptor even at very minute concentrations of transferrin in the media.[152] Evidence from peptide mapping studies and various other immunologic studies suggest that transferrin receptors of different cell types are chemically and functionally very similar. Placental and reticulocyte receptors have the same molecular weight, proteolytic digest pattern, and immune reactions.[153] Also, the mouse transferrin receptor from a T-lymphoma line E14 and C55BL/6 origin suggest a dimeric glycoprotein of 200,000 and in murine myeloma cells receptor subunits of 94,000 and 96,000 mol wt were observed.[154] Those values are very close to the 180 to 190,000 mol wt receptor observed in human tissues. This is not to say that there are not minor differences in receptors between species and even between different tissues of the same species, as demonstrated by the reactivity of certain monoclonal antibodies.[155]

Receptor affinity for transferrin by different tissues in the organism appears to be constant and this is also true for the different stages of red cell maturation;[148,152] however, the iron status of the transferrin molecule exerts an important effect, diferric transferrin having the greater affinity, monoferric transferrins intermediate affinities, and apotransferrin having no measurable affinity at a physiologic pH of 7.4.[156-158] On the other hand, at pH values of around 5, only apotransferrin forms a very stable complex with receptor.[159] As discussed later, the pH dependence of binding between the various forms of transferrin and receptor are critical to both membrane uptake and release of transferrin.[156,158-161]

B. BIOSYNTHESIS AND CATABOLISM

The biosynthesis of transferrin receptors follows a metabolic pathway that has been described for other cell surface glycoproteins.[152]

Newly formed receptors have an apparent molecular weight of 88,000. Their *in vitro* digestion with endo-β-*N*-acetyl-glucosamidase (endo H) results in the formation of a species of molecular weight of 80,000. Within 4 h, conversion into the mature form of the receptor with a molecular weight of 95,000 takes place in cultured cells. The transferrin receptor has been shown to undergo posttranslational modification (i.e., phosphorylation, acylation, glycosylation) the final form being stable against endo H digestion.[149] It has been proposed that these posttranslational modifications might be involved in directing, inserting, or anchoring of membrane receptors.[152] The receptor is released in vesicle form, a process which is likely to require membrane fusion. The released vesicles contain newly incorporated fatty acids.[150] A direct role of this acyl addition group in receptor processing during transferrin delivery appears unlikely because of the relatively slow rate of acyl group turnover.[148,162]

The half time disappearance of transferrin receptors from cells has been shown to be in the order of 2 to 3 d in NCRF-CEMT leukemia cells,[33,138] although receptors in HeLa cells have a half-life of only 14 h.[163] The extent to which receptors are degraded within cells is not clear. In developing rat and sheep reticulocytes, transferrin receptors for the most part are incorporated into vesicles and exocytosed.[164,165]

IV. INTRACELLULAR IRON DELIVERY

Early studies indicated that the half-life of transferrin in normal human circulation is about 8 d, while that of iron is only 1 to 2 h.[16,166-169] Unlike many other proteins, therefore, the transferrin survives its interaction with cells to experience 100 or more cycles of iron transport during its lifetime. The fate of transferrin and iron during the process of transferrin-mediated cellular iron uptake, however, has not been well defined until very recently.

Considerable controversy exists about the site of iron removal from these cells. It was initially believed that transferrin iron was delivered to the membrane of an immature erythroid cell and this possibility is still espoused;[141,170-172] however, a preponderance of evidence now indicates that the release of iron from transferrin occurs predominately within the cell.[54,152,159,160,173-177] Many of these studies have employed reticulocytes since it was a simple method to follow the incorporation of iron into either hemoglobin or ferritin.[128] Other cell types have also been examined with similar results.[73,175,177-182] In an energy- and temperature-dependent process, diferric and monoferric transferrin bind to transferrin receptors on the cell membrane (Figure 4). Following this, the complex is internalized in a vesicle which has been variously called an endosome or receptosome which is fused to another vesicle whose pH is less than 5.5.[183-185] The resulting acidification promotes release of iron from transferrin, and in some fashion, the released iron moves to its destination within the cell.[186,187] Lysosomes are not involved in this process, even in nonerythroid cells.[184,188] The iron-depleted transferrin remaining behind is held by its receptor at the low pH of the vesicle.[130,159,160] The apotransferrin receptor complex is then translocated to the cell membrane where the neutral pH effects release of the apotransferrin from the receptor to the plasma or surrounding solution.[160,189] There is some evidence that recycling may occur through the Golgi.[190] What makes the cycle work is the high affinity of transferrin iron for the receptor at neutral pH and the high affinity of apotransferrin for the receptor at acid pH.[73,159]

Molecular events initiating the transferrin cell cycle are not understood. Calcium and calmodulin appear to be involved in the internalization process.[191,192] It is possible that phosphorylation-dephosphorylation of the receptor plays some role in directing receptor traffic from the surface onto the endosome network and back into the surface.[164]

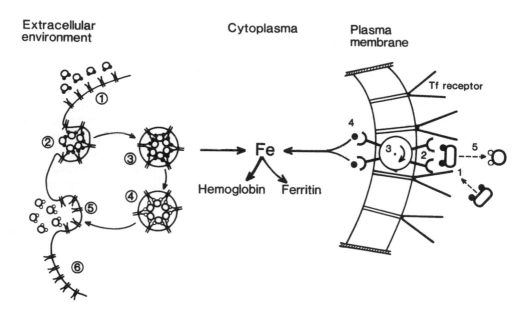

A) Receptor mediated endocytosis   **B) Stationary receptor model**

FIGURE 4.   Cellular uptake of transferrin. (A) Receptor-mediated endocytosis based on References 21, 73, 130, 159, 160: the formation of a transferrin-iron-complex at the cell membrane (1-2), its intracellular movement (2-3), iron release at pH of less than 5.5 (3-4), and subsequent return of apotransferrin to the cell membrane (4-5) is illustrated. At neutral pH, apotransferrin is released from its receptor (5). Both the released apotransferrin and the transferrin receptor can be reutilized for transport and cellular uptake of iron (6→1). (B) Stationary receptor model based on References 141, 171, 172, 214. Diferric transferrin binds to transferrin receptors on the plasma membrane (1-2), with reduction of ferric iron and release of the iron to an iron binding protein in the plasma membrane (2-3). Ferrous iron in the plasma membrane is then transported into the cytosol (3-4), where it is incorporated into hemoglobin or ferritin. Apotransferrin is then released from the receptor (5).

The integrity of the intracellular cycle may be modified by physical changes in the cell membrane which affect the ability of transferrin to react with receptor sites.[193] An increase in lipid fluidity increases the availability of transferrin receptors and a decrease in lipid fluidity decreases it by a passive mechanism.[194,195] Some modification of cellular receptor distribution in the cell may also occur. Under normal circumstances, about one third of transferrin receptors on the cell surface, the rest being in the intermediate vesicles or endosomes within the cell.[177] Treatment of human fibroblasts with epidermal growth factor results in a rapid increase in the ability of the cell membrane to bind transferrin, by accelerating the return of internalized receptors and/or retarding their internalization.[196] Treatment of macrophages with phorbol esters (PMA) or the calcium ionophore A23187 also effects the translocation of a receptor-containing compartment to the cell surface.[176] It was also reported that phorbol esters lead to the internalization of receptors even without ligands.[176]

In the developing red cell, most of the iron taken up is converted into hemoglobin within minutes.[145] An additional portion is stored as ferritin, the latter being related in amount to the transferrin saturation.[197] The extent to which the latter is available for hemoglobin synthesis is not clear, but its presence implies that the iron uptake capacity of the developing cell is in excess of that actually needed.

A. IRON EXCHANGE BEHAVIOR OF MAMMALIAN TRANSFERRIN

Much attention has been given to the interaction of transferrin iron with transferrin receptors on cell membranes to provide a supply of iron for body cells.[10,21] Biochemists have long speculated on the evolutionary advantage of the mammalian two-sited protein, and the questions of whether or not iron bound to the two sites of transferrin behaves in exactly the same way.[4] A stimulus to such studies was the report by Fletcher and Huehns[199] of nonhomogenous behavior of transferrin iron in a reticulocyte-incubation model. They suggested that one binding site preferentially delivers iron to the erythron while the other supplies nonerythroid tissues.[199] A number of supportive studies followed, some demonstrating differences in the chemical behavior of the two sites and other espousing a nonuniform iron release to reticulocytes *in vitro* and to body tissues *in vivo*.[74,200-205] Questions raised by these studies were answered only after the uptake and release of iron from the transferrin molecule were better understood.

The way that transferrin reacts with tissues to obtain iron is poorly understood. Direct contact with the unsaturated transferrin molecule is required for release of iron from RE cell to plasma since saturation of the transferrin molecule with iron interferes with this release[298] and since desferrioxamine cannot intercept iron going from the RE cell to the erythron.[206] Ascorbic acid may be required for normal mobilization of iron from tissues, and ceruloplasmin or citrate may facilitate the transfer.[207,208]

Initial attempts to determine directly the proportions of diferric and the two monoferric transferrins were carried out by urea gel electrophoresis.[209] The variable results obtained by this method may have been due to the use of iron compounds for loading which did not uniformly label binding sites[210] and iron contamination which distorted the pattern obtained from the separating system.[72,211] More detailed recent measurements of the transferrin profile after isolectric focusing and crossed immunoelectrophoresis showed a random distribution of iron on binding sites in normal human plasma under basal conditions and after *in vitro* and *in vivo* iron loading[211-213] (Figure 5). These latter findings indicate that the binding of iron to transferrin *in vivo* conforms to simple probabilistic rules, and that one atom of iron is loaded at a time.

The iron donating behavior of the transferrin molecule has also been clarified.[156,158,314 220] The two monoferric forms of transferrin have identical iron donating capacities,[158,215] both in animals and in humans.[216-218] The rate of iron donation and pattern of tissue distribution *in vivo* are identical. Iron release from transferrin to erythroid cells from either mono- or diferric transferrin is an "all or none" phenomenon leaving only apotransferrin.[216,221] While receptors cycle transferrin into the cell regardless of its iron content, there is a competitive advantage of diferric over monoferric transferrin.[156,220] Apotransferrin is not competitive. These iron-related differences in affinity between transferrin and receptor may well relate to the shape changes of the molecule during iron loading.[36,91,209] The higher affinity of the diferric molecule was responsible for the original effects described by Fletcher and Huehns.[222]

Species effects also enter into the reaction between transferrin and receptors. In homologous systems, rat reticulocyte uptake is ten times greater than that of the homologous system of human transferrin and reticulocytes, but this may simply relate to a different receptor number on the reticulocytes of the two species. However, differences do exist in the capacity of transferrins and receptors of different species to interact. In general, homologous transferrins donate at a faster rate as compared to heterologous transferrins. In some instances, delivery between species is very limited, as exemplified by the delivery of iron from fetal calf transferrin to human reticulocytes.[223] Transferrins from eutherian mammals donate iron to noneutherian mammals with a facility nearly equal to that of the homologous protein.[224] On the other hand, transferrin from noneutherian species with few exceptions cannot donate iron to cells from eutherian mammals.

Iron binding from fragments corresponding to the N- and C-terminal domains of transferrin produced by trypsin and thermolysin digestion are variably affected. Trypsin digestion considerably reduces the ability of bovine transferrins to donate iron to rabbit reticulocytes, slightly reduces the iron donation of rabbit transferrin fragments, and has almost no effect on iron donation by humans or horse transferrin fragments.[225]

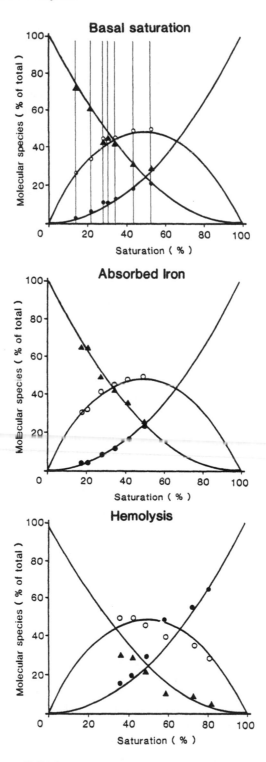

FIGURE 5.   Separation of apo, monoferric, and diferric transferrin as a function of transferrin saturation in normal subjects. Distribution was random under basal conditions, during iron absorption and with hemolysis. (From Huebers, H. A., Josephson, B., Huebers, E., Csiba, E., and Finch, C. A., *Proc. Natl. Acad. Sci. U.S.A.*, 81, 4326, 1984. With permission.)

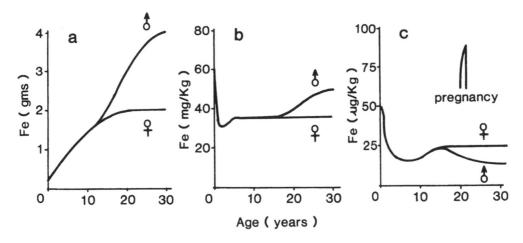

FIGURE 6. Iron balance as a function of age. Panel A shows the increase in total body iron, panel B the body iron concentration, and panel C, the amount absorption required to maintain iron balance and (in the case of pregnancy) to meet fetal requirements. (From Bothwell, T. H., Charlton, R. W., Cook, J. D., and Finch, C. A., *Iron Metabolism in Man,* Blackwell Scientific, Oxford, 1979. With permission.)

V. PATHWAYS OF IRON EXCHANGE

A. IRON BALANCE

Iron balance involves iron requirements on the one hand and iron absorption on the other. Human iron requirements include, more specifically, needs for growth and replacement of physiologic losses and uterine losses due to menstruation and pregnancy (Figure 6). Physiological iron losses from the body include acute bleeding from the intestine, iron in bile, exfoliation of iron-containing mucosal cells from the intestine, urinary iron, and skin desquamation.[226] All together, these losses represent about 1 mg/d in the adult male and can be reduced to 0.5 mg in the iron-deficient individual and less than 0.1 mg in the infant.[227] The mucosal absorptive mechanism compensates for any less favorable iron balance by increasing absorption, but restrictions are given by the availability of food iron. After initial solubilization of available iron by gastric acid, most of the iron entering the small bowel is absorbed in the upper duodenum. When more alkaline pH is reached in the upper jejunum, iron is complexed to mucosal transferrin in the lumen and absorbed. Another system exists for the absorption of hemoglobin iron.[228-230] These mechanisms act in concert to procure iron. It appears that the first step in absorption, i.e., membrane uptake is the most important point of regulation.[231-233]

The way iron gets through the mucosa has not been defined, but it has been apparent for some time that absorption is regulated and is more important than iron excretion in determining body iron balance. Investigators spoke of a "mucosal block".[226] These became identified with mucosal ferritin, since a strong inverse relationship was observed between mucosal ferritin content and the amount of iron absorbed. The principal physiologic parameters influencing iron uptake are previous dietary exposure, the amount of storage iron within the body, and erythropoiesis.[226,227,234,235]

B. BODY IRON

Body iron of the healthy mature newborn is about 250 to 280 mg.[236,237] This is about 6% of the total iron content of the adult. In the infant, about 75% of the iron can be found in hemoglobin, 10% in the myoglobin and tissue enzymes, and about 15% stored as ferritin and hemosiderin, principally in the reticuloendothelial cells and hepatocytes.[238] Corresponding values for the adult are depicted in Table 1. Iron requirements are proportional to the

TABLE 1
Human Body Iron (70-kg male)

	mg	Total (%)
Hemoglobin	2600	65.0
Ferritin	450	11.2
Hemosiderin	400	10.0
Nonheme enzymes	400	10.0
Myoglobin	138	3.5
Cytochromes	8	0.2
Transferrin	4	0.1
Total body iron	4000	100.0

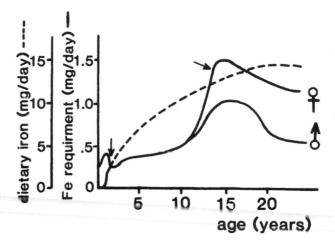

FIGURE 7.   Changes in iron requirement from birth until the completion of growth (continuous black line) in girls and in boys. The broken line indicates the iron content of the diet. Arrows point to the two critical period life where an iron deficiency anemia of a purely nutritional type can be expected. (From Bothwell, T. H., Charlton, R. W., Cook, J. D., and Finch, C. A., *Iron Metabolism in Man*, Blackwell Scientific, Oxford, 1979. With permission.)

weight increase. One kilogram of weight is associated with 35 to 45 mg of iron requirement. A 7-kg weight increase in the first year of life requires about 280 mg of iron, i.e., a daily requirement of 0.7 to 0.8 μg.[239] The high hemoglobin of 20 g/dl at birth and early destruction of excess red cells supplement the supply of iron for the growing infant for about the first 4 to 5 months. Thereafter the iron stores of most infants are exhausted. Consequently, there is a tendency to develop iron deficiency anemia of a true nutritional type (Figure 7). After the first year, the rate of body growth slows down and is relatively steady between the 2nd and 11th year of life. It is then followed by an adolescent growth spurt that is particularly rapid between 11 and 14 years in the case of girls, and 14 to 17 years in boys.[240] It is during adolescence that the male and female part company with respect to iron balance. The male enjoys a highly favorable position once growth is complete, needing only 1 mg of iron or less to replace physiological blood losses.[241] In the adult female, there is an additional requirement of about 0.5 mg/d due to menstruation.[240,242]

These developmental changes in iron requirement are also reflected by the size of total storage iron. Total storage iron may be determined directly from the amount of iron that is mobilized by phlebotomy, but the more practical method for clinical purposes is measurement

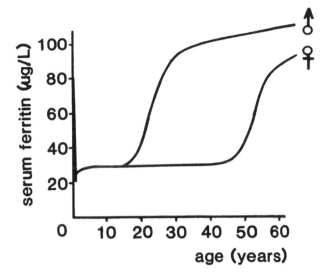

FIGURE 8. Serum ferritin levels according to sex and age. The serum ferritin reflects the marrow stores of the individual; however, the pattern of the serum ferritin level will depend on the sex and the age of the individual. Before age 20, the serum ferritin level is usually between 20 and 40 μg/l. During the adult years, the values for males rise progressively during the early adult years to reach levels of about 100 μg/l. In contrast, most women remain between 20 and 40 μg/l throughout their child-bearing years and increase only after menopause. (From Bothwell, T. H., Charlton, R. W., Cook, J. D., and Finch, C. A., *Iron Metabolism in Man*, Blackwell Scientific, Oxford, 1979. With permission.)

of serum ferritin. Serum ferritin, which appears to be secreted from all ferritin producing body cells, differs from tissue ferritin in that the former is partly glycosylated and almost free of iron.[5] The amount of ferritin protein in circulating blood parallels the concentrations of storage iron within the body wherever that iron may be.[243] In the normal adult, 1 μg of ferritin is roughly equivalent to 8 mg of storage iron, provided inflammation has been excluded.[243] However, a more accurate approach, and one that is essential in infants and children, is to express a relationship between ferritin and stores on a per kilogram basis.[240] Ferritin at 1 μg is equivalent to 120 μg iron per kilogram. There is a rapid change in serum ferritin concentration during the first month after birth and the levels decline from about 100 μg/l at 1 month to levels of only about 30 μg/l. The ferritin levels remain low from the age of 6 months to about 15 years and in women this level is maintained until menopause (Figure 8).

C. IRON DISTRIBUTION

Once iron gains access to the body interior, it is bound by transferrin and distributed to body tissues. While 3 to 5% of iron passing through the plasma comes from absorption in the adult human, as much as 30% of plasma iron may be derived from an iron-fortified diet in the human infant.[244] Most of the iron transferred in the body, however, is not derived from absorption, but results from the release of iron from the hemoglobin of effete red cells and the acquisition by apotransferrin of this iron (Figure 9). Iron transferrin, whether the iron is obtained from the gut or from the reticuloendothelial system, is largely directed to the bone marrow where the iron is then delivered to hemoglobin-synthesizing erythroid cells finishing up in mature erythrocytes.[245,246] Perhaps 80 to 90% of the iron traffic borne by transferrin is destined for hemoglobin synthesis.[247] While this movement of iron from eryth-

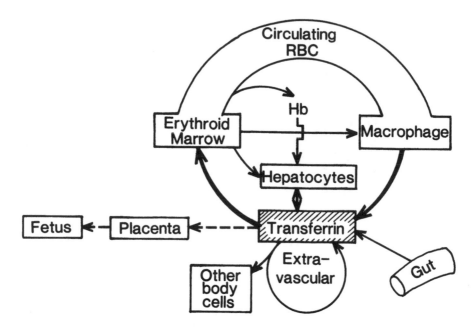

FIGURE 9.   Pathways of human internal iron exchange. Transferrin iron incorporated into the developing red cells (and delivered to the fetus via the placenta) circulates for the most part of the lifespan of the red cell. Thereafter effete cells are catabolized in the RE cell. Some wastage iron from immature erythroid cells is processed by the RE cell and some free hemoglobin is processed by the hepatocyte.

roid precursors to the circulation within red cells and later to reticuloendothelial cells constitutes the major portion of erythroid iron turnover, some red cell iron short circuits the circulating red cell mass.[2] In the process of hemoglobin formation, some erythrocyte iron is deposited as ferritin and this form of nonheme iron is removed from the red cell and is processed by the reticuloendothelial cells of the marrow or spleen. In addition, there is a small fraction of hemoglobin iron lost with enucleation or from intravascular breakdown of circulating red cells which combines with haptoglobin in the plasma and is cleared by the hepatocyte.[248,249] These various red cell pathways are subject to change with expansion or contraction of the red cell marrow and particularly with increased red cell destruction during maturation or in circulation.

The importance of transferrin for iron exchange is perhaps best explained in the very rare genetic disorder known as atransferrinemia.[250-254] The paradoxical situation in atransferrinemia is that there is, on the one hand, generalized iron overload and, on the other hand, a profound and refractory hypochromic, microcytic anemia due to an inadequate iron supply.[251,253] Without transferrin it is difficult to get iron into cells for the biosynthesis of hemoglobin and it is equally difficult to regulate the absorption of iron.[2] In the presence of transferrin, the most relevant biological expression of iron supply is the transferrin saturation because of the direct relationship between saturation and diferric iron and the much greater capacity of diferric transferrin to deliver iron to tissues[255,256] (Figure 10). Normal saturation cycles between 35% in the morning and 20% at night, but occasionally will go as low as 15% and as high as 50% or even higher. Such fluctuations are not surprising in view of the small amount of plasma iron in relation to the amount of iron required by tissues. Similar saturation levels are seen from adolescence to old age. In the presence of basal erythropoiesis, a saturation of 16% or more delivers an adequate amount of iron for tissue requirements. When the transferrin saturation is less than 16%, hemoglobin synthesis can no longer be sustained at a basal level, causing iron-deficient erythropoiesis. The fall in percent saturation

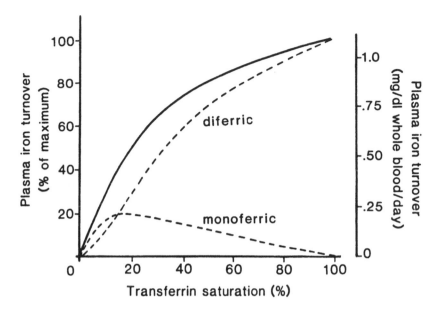

FIGURE 10. Effect of transferrin saturation on plasma iron turnover. The calculated contribution of iron uptake from the diferric and monoferric transferrin pool of the plasma is indicated.

may be due to either an absolute deficiency of iron or an inflammatory state; however, the patterns of plasma iron and total iron-binding capacity are usually quite different in these two conditions. Patients with absolute iron deficiency tend to have a higher than normal TIBC (that is, transferrin level), while inflammation is associated with a decrease in the total iron-binding capacity. High percent saturation (greater than 60%) is occasionally seen as normal fluctuation, but persistence of this deviation usually signals hepatic disease, abnormal erythropoiesis, or parenchymal iron overload (Figure 11).

Iron supplied to transferrin in infancy and childhood has presented a problem of interpretation. Transferrin saturation is lower than in adulthood and often falls below the critical level of 16% established in the adult.[257-259] Other indices of iron status, including red cell protoporphyrin and ferritin, also show values that would indicate iron deficiency in the adult. However, iron therapy does not necessarily improve the hemoglobin concentration as would be expected in an iron-deficient adult. It has, therefore, been suggested that these findings constitute a physiologic difference in the regulation of iron supply in childhood, one resembling to some degree the changes produced by inflammation (Table 2). Criteria for identification of iron deficiency at different ages employed in the NHANES II survey are summarized in the accompanying table (Table 2).

Another cellular exchange is between transferrin and the hepatocyte[247,260] (Table 3). In contrast to the mononuclear macrophage, which is only able to receive iron from senescent red cells, the hepatocyte can receive iron from plasma transferrin; however, both types of cells can donate iron to plasma transferrin. If plasma iron falls to iron depletion, the hepatocyte releases iron, whereas with an increase of plasma transferrin saturation, there is an increased net flow into its ferritin or hemosiderin stores. One other aspect of hepatocyte iron exchange which is unique among body cells is the ability to take up nontransferrin iron from the plasma. Iron citrate or ascorbate injected intravenously in the transferrin saturated organism or iron absorbed from intestine in excess of iron tranferrin binding capacity is rapidly removed from circulation by the hepatocytes.[261,262]

The other efficient system of iron uptake is seen in pregnancy. Iron uptake by the fetus and growth are roughly in parallel and in proportion to each other. This is achieved by the

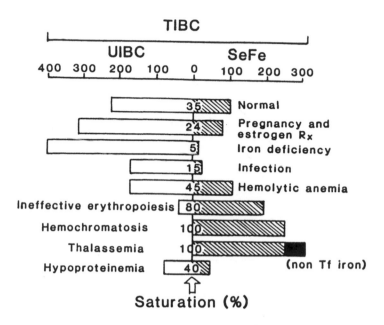

FIGURE 11. Transferrin and its iron. The serum iron in a normal individual ranges from 50 to 150 µg/dl of plasma, with 100 µg/dl being an average normal value. This represents only about 1/3 of the binding capacity of transferrin so that the saturation (%) is about 30%. Both the serum iron and the total iron-binding capacity level are altered by disease states. Pregnancy is associated with a modest reduction in the serum iron and an increase in the total iron-binding capacity. Iron deficiency shows an even more striking change with a major reduction in the serum iron and a dramatic increase in the total iron-binding capacity, giving a percent saturation below 10%. In contrast, infection reduces both the serum iron and the total iron-binding capacity. The pattern observed with most hemolytic anemias is quite different from that observed with marked ineffective erythropoiesis. In the hemolytic anemias, the plasma iron is relatively normal, while with ineffective erythropoiesis there may be an increase in the serum iron with near total saturation of the iron-binding capacity. A similar pattern is seen with hemochromatosis. Severe starvation, nephrotic syndrome, and chronic inflammatory disease can result in marked hypoproteinemia with pronounced reductions in transferrin.

placenta developing transferrin receptors and the number of receptors is the main factor accounting for the changing rate of iron transfer through the placenta during growth.[263] The receptor-rich placenta can successfully compete with the erythroid marrow for transferrin, and the iron taken up is rapidly passed on to fetal transferrin and deposited in fetal tissues. As pregnanacy progresses and the fetus is enlarged, about 20% of maternal plasma iron turnover goes to the fetus (Figure 12). The iron of the fetus is mainly accumulated during the last few weeks of interuterine life (Figure 12). In the human, the requirement of the fetus is about 8.8% of body iron over 280 d.[264] The maximum amount of iron transferred 1 d is about 7 mg or 0.3% of maternal iron. These requirements of the human fetus are such that they can probably be met by uptake of iron from the plasma, regardless of the degree of hyperferemia in the mother;[265,266] however, a mother will become that much more iron depleted. This is borne out by many studies in which hemoglobin concentrations of newborn children have been shown to be unchanged by iron deficiency in the mother, and ferritin concentrations of the fetal serum reflecting iron stores have been shown to be little affected by maternal iron deficiency.[267,268] It is noteworthy that the plasma iron level of Bantu women does not decrease significantly during pregnancy and they usually do not develop anemia, presumably because of the high iron content of the diet.[269] The decrease

TABLE 2
Indicators of Iron Deficiency

Test	Infant	Child	Adult
Plasma ferritin (μg/l)	—	<10	<12
Transferrin saturation (%)	<12	<14	<16
RBC protoporphrin (μg/dl)	>80	>75	>70
Mean rbc volume (fl)	<73	<76	<80

TABLE 3
Iron Deficient Erythropoiesis

	Transferrin level (μg/dl)	Saturation (%)	Ferritin (μg/l)	Iron stores
Iron deficiency	350—500	5—12	<12	Absent
Inflammation	150—300	<16	>100	Present

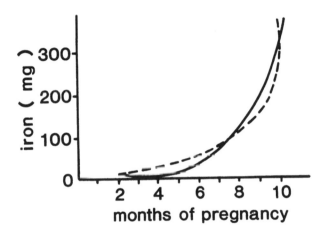

FIGURE 12.   Increase in the iron content in the human fetus during pregnancy. Solid line: Iob and Swanson, broken line Jerlow. (Iron loss and iron requirement in *Iron Metabolism*, Bernat, I., Ed., Plenum Press, New York, 1983, 129.)

in plasma iron observed in pregnant women not taking iron may be ascribed only partly to iron depletion, and occurs as a consequence of the expanded red cell mass and fetal iron requirements.[265-268] The conspicuous increase in TIBC to over 400 μg/dl is due in part to iron depletion, but hormonal effects have been shown to be additionally involved.[270]

VI. PATHOPHYSIOLOGY OF IRON EXCHANGE

Some insight into the pathophysiology of iron exchange is provided by the distribution of iron stores. In the normal adult, about two thirds of the reserve iron supply is held by RE cells and about one third by hepatocytes. RE cells occupy the most prominent position, supplying perhaps two thirds of the iron passing through the plasma. Within the RE cell, there is a constantly changing distribution of processed iron between storage vs. return of iron to transferrin.[271,272] When more iron is acquired for red cell production, an increased amount of processed iron is returned at once to transferrin and in addition, storage iron is mobilized. The hepatocyte acts as a regulator of plasma iron by taking up increased amounts in hyperferremic states or mobilizing stores to supply increased iron to transferrin in situations

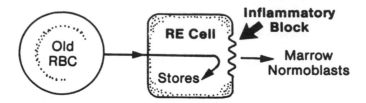

FIGURE 13.   Reticuloendothelial iron blockade with inflammation. The iron recovered from the destruction of old red cells accumulates within the reticuloendothelial cells because of an inflammatory block directed at release of iron to circulating transferrin. (From Hilman, R. S. and Finch, C. A., *Red Cell Manual,* 5th ed., F. A. Davis, Philadelphia, 1985, 1. With permission.)

where requirements are increased. At equilibrium, the release of iron to transferrin by the liver is greater than its uptake, since the liver is also receiving iron from plasma in the form of haptoglobin-hemoglobin complex (Figure 9).

These two storage areas ordinarily respond together to the needs of the various body tissues for iron, particularly those of the erythron, but differences emerge in various pathologic states. In infection, RE stores appear disproportionately enlarged, even though iron released from both RE cells and hepatocytes is impaired (Figure 13), presumably due to the greater rate of accumulation in the RE cell.[273] RE stores also predominate in patients with aplastic anemia who are repeatedly transfused and in the South African Black ingesting alcoholic beverages of high iron content.[2,274] Parenchymal iron overload is seen in the two genetic disorders most commonly associated with idiopathic hemochromatosis and thalassemia.[2,275,276] Despite differences in underlying defects, source of excess iron, rate of iron accumulation, and life expectancy, both disorders are associated with similar tissue changes (skin pigmentation, hepatomegaly, endocrine abnormalities, and most notably involvement of the heart). Removal of excess iron is of the utmost importance in the management of both diseases.

Idiopathic hemochromatosis is a rare HLA-related disorder of body iron regulation.[275,277] In the individual homozygous for this gene, there is an increased iron absorption from the gastrointestinal tract and a failure of the reticuloendothelial system to retain iron.[277,278] The iron overload (about 20 to 40 g) can easily be eradicated by phlebotomy.[277-279] Reversal of cardiac failure and improvement in liver function with iron removal demonstrates the toxic nature of the iron deposits.[277,278]

Thalassemia major clearly poses a health problem in many countries and can be regarded as a prototype of the iron loading anemias.[279,280] These diseases present a triple problem, namely severe anemia, massive enlargement of the erythroid marrow, and iron overload. Until recently, the outlook in thalassemia major was poor.[279,281,282] Death of chronically ill children occurred often in the first decade. Those who survived longer were dwarfed and sexually immature, and those who did not die of incidental infection almost invariably succumbed to cardiac failure due to myocardial siderosis.[280,282] An advance in the management was the recurrent blood transfusion of the thalassemic child. This reversed skeletal abnormalities and permitted normal development until adolescence. Central to this improvement was the suppression of erythropoiesis which normalized bone vs. bone marrow relationships, blood flow distribution through the body, and reduced iron absorption.[277-279] However, the iron overload, previously the result of increased iron absorption, was now more than supplanted by the transfused red cell iron, amounting to about 1 mg/kg/d.[2,280,281] Sexual maturation of transfused patients was still arrested but now because of the toxic effects of iron. The majority of the children died by the third decade due to iron overload.[280] With the inability to remove the damaging iron by phlebotomy, there was growing interest in some form of chelator therapy which might reduce the effects of iron in these individuals.[279,281,283-285]

TABLE 4
Properties of the Ideal Iron Chelating Agent

1. It must be efficient and selective for chelating Fe^{3+}.
2. Iron removal should be from parenchymal tissues at risk of toxic damage, and the chelate should be able to bind avidly to iron in competition with transferrin.
3. After iron is chelated, it should be promptly excreted in a nontoxic form through urine and/or bile.
4. During the process of iron excretion, there must be no redistribution of iron from nontoxic storage depots to more vulnerable tissues, such as the heart.
5. The ideal chelating drug should be inexpensive.
6. The drug should be orally effective to reduce the problems of compliance.
7. The ideal drug should have no immediate or long-term toxicity.
8. The ideal drug should permit a net removal of iron from patients with preexistent iron overload and prevent iron buildup and related tissue damage in patients at risk of iron overload.

TABLE 5
Modalities of Administration of Desferrioxamine B

Intermittent intramuscular injection:	500 to 750 mg, in 2 to 4 ml H_2O
Continuous infusion technique:[a]	
Intravenous:	By drip, over 10 h, in 1/3 normal saline
Subcutaneous:	By continuous infusion, over 10 h, in 5.5 ml H_2O (with or without 11 mg hydrocortisone), administered over 10 h with a syringe pump attached under the patient's slipper, through a no. 25 butterfly needle inserted in the calf or in the skin of the abdomen

[a] The total dose of desferrioxamine to be given is best determined for each patient individually by performing a dose-response curve. In most older patients, the optimal dose is in the range of 2 to 4 g/d or about 25 to 40 mg/kg. This dose leads to urinary excretion of 20 to 90 mg/d. Similar amounts may be excreted in the feces.

Iron chelation therapy was started some 20 years ago in patients with iron overload and anemia.[2] At the present time, the ideal chelating agent (Table 4) has still to be found and only one drug has been judged to be clinically useful. Desferrioxamine B, a siderophore produced by *Streptomyces pilosus*, forms a very stable complex with iron but not with other metal ions, is effective *in vivo*, and has few side effects. The initial therapy with daily intramuscular bolus injections of desferrioxamine proved insufficient to prevent iron loading in the face of frequent repeated transfusions. Since the half-time of desferrioxamine in the circulation is only 5 to 10 min, it must be administered by continuous infusion to be effective. The required amount of desferrioxamine B (usually 2 to 4 g/d) is most conveniently given with a small portable infusion pump.[286-288] If significant amounts are given over sufficient time, they have been shown to result in negative iron balance in patients with thalassemia with any level of iron loading (Table 5). Concomitant ascorbic acid treatment in ascorbate depleted individuals appears to render tissue more accessible to desferrioxamine, although the effect may be more limited when both urinary and stool iron excretion are taken into account. Unfortunately, ascorbic acid also appears to enchance the toxicity of tissue iron. Deterioration of heavily iron-loaded patients is well documented.[2,279] For this reason, ascorbic acid should be given in limited amounts (100 to 200 mg/d) only to individuals who are ascorbic acid depleted.

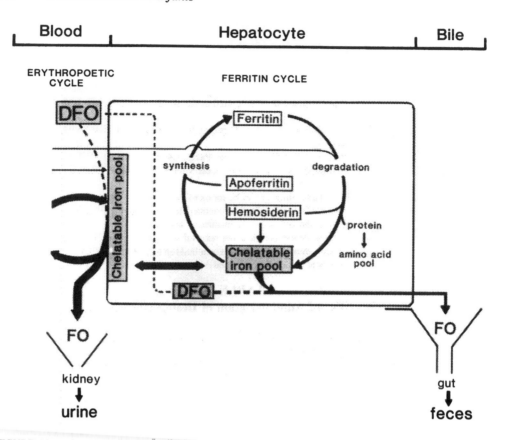

FIGURE 14.   Alternate pathways for the removal of hepatocyte iron by desferrioxamine. Urinary iron relates to the competition between transferrin and chelate at the hepatocyte membrane and is a function of the activity of the erythron. The iron excreted in the feces is derived from an intracellular pool related to the anabolic/catabolic cycle of the ferritin/hemosiderin system. Obstruction to biliary radicles as may occur in cirrhosis appears to divert biliary chelated iron into the urine. (From Huebers, H. A., *Blut*, 47, 61, 1983. With permission.)

The greater efficiency of continuous infusion is thought to be due to a constant exposure of a labile iron pool to a chelating agent. Recent studies have emphasized the importance of the hepatocyte as the locus of iron chelation by desferrioxamine and have discounted earlier studies suggesting macrophage stores as the site of primary chelate attack.[289,290] Desferrioxamine enters the hepatocyte (whereas ferrioxamine cannot), loads with iron, and ferrioxamine is excreted in the bile (Figure 14). The principal intrahepatic pool tapped by the chelate appears to be related to ferritin and hemosiderin. Chelate action probably takes place at the time these molecules are degraded and before iron is reinserted into a new molecule.[276,283,289,291] The yield from this pool relates to the amount of chelate which enters the hepatocyte and the size of the pool present. Given sufficient chelate dosage, this pathway, which results in iron excretion in the stool, represents the largest single fraction of iron excretion in individuals with parenchymal iron overload.[277,279,283] Iron chelate excretion, however, also occurs in the urine. This second pool of chelatable iron is related to erythropoiesis activity.[283] There is some evidence that this pool relates to the competition between transferrin and chelate at the hepatocyte membrane.[276,283] Of further interest is the relationship between these two chelatable pools. When erythropoiesis is stimulated, the reverse occurs.[276,283]

Recent advances in the technique for the administration of desferrioxamine by subcutaneous infusion leaves no doubt that regular treatment by such a regimen can establish negative iron balance in transfusion-dependent patients. The problem is the cost and difficulty of parenteral administration in normalizing iron balance with DFO. Future developments and treatment of patients with iron overload by chelating agents will depend on the solution of a number of problems, particularly the developments of an orally effective agent of low toxicity and cost which can be given prophylactically.[292] This is all the more important since there is increasing evidence that increased intestinal iron absorption is a major contributor to early death in thalassemia intermedia where transfusion therapy is usually not given.

REFERENCES

1. **Frieden, E.**, The biochemical evolution of the iron and copper proteins, in *Trace Element Metabolism in Animals*, 2nd ed., Hoekstra, W. G. et al., Eds., University Park Press, Baltimore, 1974, 105.
2. **Bothwell, T. H., Charlton, R. W., Cook, J. D., and Finch, C. A.**, *Iron Metabolism in Man*, Blackwell Scientific, Oxford, 1979.
3. **Holland, H. D.**, *The Chemical Evolution of the Atmosphere and Oceans*, Princeton University Press, Princeton, N. J., 1984.
4. **Aisen, P. and Listowsky, I.**, Iron transport and storage proteins, *Annu. Rev. Biochem.*, 49, 357, 1980.
5. **Worwood, M.**, Serum ferritin, in *Iron in Biochemistry and Medicine II*, Jacobs, A. and Worwood, M., Eds., Academic Press, London, 1980, 203.
6. **Bezkorovainy, A.**, Absorption of nonheme iron, in *Biochemistry of Nonheme Iron*, Frieden, E., Ed., Plenum Press, New York, 1980, 47.
7. **Neilands, J. B.**, Microbial iron compounds, *Annu. Rev. Biochem.*, 50, 713, 1981.
8. **Finch, C. A.**, Body iron exchange in man, *J. Clin. Invest.*, 38, 392, 1959.
9. **Aisen, P. and Brown, E. B.**, Structure and function of transferrin, *Prog. Hematol.*, 14, 31, 1977.
10. **Aisen, P. and Brown, E. B.**, The iron-binding function of transferrin, *Prog. Hematol.*, 9, 25, 1975.
11. **Munro, H. N.**, Evolution of protein metabolism in mammals, in *Mammalian Protein Metabolism*, Academic Press, New York, 1969, 133.
12. **Pippard, M. J. and Weatherall, D. J.**, Iron absorption in non-transfused iron loading anaemias: prediction of risk for iron loading and response to iron chelation treatment in B thalassaemia intermedia and congenital sideroblastic anaemias, *Haematology*, 17, 2, 1984.
13. **Pootrakul, P., Huebers, H., Finch, C., Pippard, M., and Cazzola, M.**, Iron metabolism in thalassemia, *Proc. Int. Cong. Thalassemia*, 2, 1986.
14. **Milder, M., Cook, J. D., Stray, S., and Finch, C. A.**, Idiopathic hemochromatosis, an interim report, *Medicine*, 59, 34, 1980.
15. **Stein, M., Blayney, D., Feit, T., et al.**, Acute iron poisoning in children, *West. J. Med.*, 125, 289, 1976.
16. **Cromwell, S. M.**, The metabolism of transferrin, in *Protides of the Biological Fluids*, Peeters, H., Ed., Elsevier, Amsterdam, 1963, 484.
17. **Martin, A. W., Huebers, E., Huebers, H., Webb, J., and Finch, C. A.**, A mono-sited transferrin from a representative deuterostoms, *Blood*, 64, 1048, 1984.
18. **Huebers, H. and Finch, C. A.**, Transferrin: physiological behavior and clinical implications, *Blood*, 64, 763, 1984.
19. **Schade, A. L. and Caroline, L.**, An iron-binding component in human blood plasma, *Science*, 104, 340, 1946.
20. **Laurell, C. and Ingelman, B.**, The iron-binding protein of swine serum, *Acta Chem. Scand.*, 1, 770, 1947.
21. **Morgan, E. H.**, Transferrin, biochemistry, physiology and clinical significance, in *Molecular Aspects of Medicine*, Pergamon Press, Oxford, 1981, 1.
22. **Aisen, P.**, Transferrin metabolism and the liver, *Semin. Liver Dis.*, 4, 192, 1984.
23. **Mazurier, J., Metz-Boutigue, M., Jolles, J., Spik, G., Montreuil, J., and Jolles, P.**, Human lacto-transferrin: molecular, functional, and evolutionary comparisons with human serum transferrin and hen ovo tranferrin, *Experientia*, 39, 135, 1983.
24. **Chasteen, N. D.**, Transferrin: a perspective, in *Advances in Inorganic Biochemistry*, Vol. 5, Theil, E., Eichhorn, G. L., and Marzilli, L., Eds., Elsevier, New York, 1983, 202.
25. **Giblett, E. R.**, Transferrin, *Physiol. Pharmacol.*, 5, 555, 1974.
26. **Williams, J.**, The evolution of transferrin, *Trends Biochem. Sci.*, 7, 394, 1982.

27. **Lane, R. S.,** Transferrin, in *Structure and Function of Plasma Proteins,* 2nd ed., Allison, A. C., Ed., Plenum Press, New York, 1976, 53.
28. **Nemet, K. and Simonovits, I.,** The biological role of lactoferrin, *Haematologia,* 18, 3, 1985.
29. **Metz-Boutigue, M.-H., Jolles, J., Mazurier, J., et al.,** Structural studies concerning human lactotransferrin: its relatedness with human serum transferrin and evidence for internal homology, *Biochime,* 60, 557, 1978.
30. **Hu, H.-Y. Y. and Aisen, P.,** Molecular characteristics of the transferrin-receptor complex of the rabbit reticulocyte, *J. Supramol. Struct.,* 8, 349, 1978.
31. **Larrick, J. W. and Cresswell, P.,** Transferrin receptors on human B and T lymphoblastoid cell lines, *Biochem. Biophys. Acta,* 583, 483, 1979.
32. **Newman, R., Schneider, C., and Sutherland, R., et al.,** The transferrin receptor, *Trends Biochem. Sci.,* 7, 397, 1982.
33. **Testa, U.,** Transferrin receptors: structure and function, *Curr. Topics Hematol.,* 5, 127, 1985.
34. **Davies, M., Parry, J. E., and Sutcliffe, R. G.,** Examination of different preparations of human placental plasma membrane for the binding of insulin, transferrin and immunoglobulins, *J. Reprod. Fertil.,* 63, 315, 1981.
35. **Charlwood, P. A.,** Differential sedimentation-velocity and gel-filtration measurements on human apotransferrin and iron-transferrin, *Biochem. J.,* 125, 1019, 1971.
36. **Charlwood, P. A.,** Comparison of the sedimentation and gel-filtration behaviour of human apotransferrin and its copper and iron complexes, *Biochem. J.,* 133, 749, 1973.
37. **MacGillivray, R. T. A., Mendez, E., Shewale, J. G., Sinha, S., Lineback-Zins, J., and Brew, K.,** The primary structure of human serum transferrin, *J. Biol. Chem.,* 258, 3543, 1983.
38. **Uzan, G., Frain, M., Park, I., et al.,** Molecular cloning and sequence analysis of cDNA for human transferrin, *Biochem. Biophys. Res. Commun.,* 119, 273, 1984.
39. **Gorinsky, B., Horsburg, C., Lindley, P. F., et al.,** Evidence for the bilobe of nature of diferric rabbit plasma, *Nature,* 281, 157, 1979.
40. **Abola, J. E., Wood, M. K., Chweh, A., Abraham, D., and Pulsinelli, P. D.,** Structure of hen ovotransferrin at 5 Å resolution, in *The Biochemistry and Physiology of Iron,* Saltman, P. and Hegenauer, J., Eds., Elsevier/North Holland, Amsterdam, 1982, 27.
41. **Jeltsch, J. and Chambon, P.,** The complete nucleotide sequence of the chick ovotransferrin mRNA, *Eur. J. Biochem.,* 122, 291, 1982.
42. **MacGillivray, R. T. A., Mendez, E., Sinha, S. K., et al.,** The complete amino acid sequence of human serum transferrin, *Proc. Natl. Acad. Sci. U.S.A.,* 79, 2504, 1982.
43. **Spik, G. and Mazurier, J.,** Comparative structural and conformational studies of polypeptide chain, carbohydrate moiety and binding sites of human serotransferrin and lactotransferrin, in *Proteins of Iron Metabolism,* Brown, E. B., Aisen, P., Fielding, J., and Crichton, R. R., Eds., Grune & Stratton, New York, 1977, 143.
44. **Williams, J., Ellerman, T. C., Kingston, I. B., Wilkins, A. C., and Kuhn, K. A.,** The primary structure of hen ovotransferrin, *Eur. J. Biochem.,* 122, 297, 1982.
45. **Park, I., Schaeffer, E. L., Alessandro, S., Baralle, F. E., and Cohen, G. N.,** Organization of the human transferrin gene: direct evidence that it orginated by gene duplication, *Proc. Natl. Acad. Sci. U.S.A.,* 82, 3149, 1985.
46. **Yang, F., Lum, J. B., McGill, J. R., et al.,** Human transferrin: cDNA characterization and chromosomal localization, *Proc. Natl. Acad. Sci. U.S.A.,* 81, 2752, 1984.
47. **Chasteen, N. D.,** The identification of the probable locus of iron and anion binding in the transferrins, *Trends Biochem. Sci.,* 8, 272, 1983.
48. **Luk, C. K.,** Study of the nature of the metal-binding sites and estimate of the distance between the metal-binding sites in transferrin using trivalent lanthanide ions as fluorescent probes, *Biochemistry,* 10, 2838, 1971.
49. **Meares, C. F. and Ledbetter, J. E.,** Energy transfer between terbium and iron bound to transferrin: reinvestigation of the distance between metal-binding sites, *Biochemistry,* 16, 5178, 1977.
50. **Aisen, P., Leibman, A., and Pinkowitz, R. A.,** The anion-binding functions of transferrin, *Adv. Exp. Med. Biol.,* 48, 125, 1974.
51. **Schlabach, M. R. and Bates, G. W.,** The synergistic binding of anions and Fe^{3+} by transferrin, *J. Biol. Chem.,* 250, 2182, 1975.
52. **Egyed, A.,** The significance of transferrin-bound bicarbonate in the uptake of iron by reticulocytes, *Biochim. Biophys. Acta,* 304, 805, 1973.
53. **Schulman, H. N., Martinez-Medellin, J., and Sidloi, R.,** The reticulocyte-mediated release of iron and bicarbonate from transferrin: effect of metabolic inhibitors, *Biochim. Biophys. Acta,* 343, 529, 1974.
54. **Octave, J.-N., Schneider, Y.-J., Trouet, A., et al,** Iron uptake and utilization by mammalian cells, I. Cellular uptake of transferrin and iron, *Trends Biochem. Sci.,* 8, 217, 1983.
55. **Aisen, P., Aasa, R., and Redfield, A. G.,** The chromium, manganese and cobalt complexes of transferrin, *J. Biol. Chem.,* 244, 4628, 1969.

56. **Beamish, M. R. and Brown, E. B.,** A comparison of the behavior of ^{111}In and ^{59}Fe-labelled transferrin on incubation with human and rat reticulocytes, *Blood,* 43, 703, 1974.

57. **Evans, R. W., Donovan, J. W., and Williams, J.,** Calorimetric studies on the binding of iron and aluminum to the amino- and carboxyl-terminal fragments of hen ovotransferrin, *FEBS Lett.,* 83, 19, 1977.

58. **Lau, S.-J. and Sarkar, B.,** Comparative studies of manganese (II)-, nickel (II)-, zinc(II)-, cadmium(II)-, and iron(III)-binding components in human cord and adult sera, *Can. J. Biochem. Cell Biol.,* 62, 449, 1984.

59. **O'Hara, P. B. and Bersohn, R.,** Resolution of the two metal binding sites of human serum transferrin by low-temperature excitation of bound europium(III), *Biochemistry,* 21, 5269, 1982.

60. **Sabbioni, E., Rade, J., and Bertolero, F.,** Relationships between iron and vanadium metabolism: the exchange of vanadium between transferrin and ferritin, *J. Inorg. Biochem.,* 12, 307, 1980.

61. **Woodworth, R. C.,** The mechanism of metal binding to conalbumin and siderophilin, *Protides Biol. Fluids,* 14, 37, 1966.

62. **Beamish, M. R. and Brown, E. B.,** The metabolism of transferrin-bound [111]In ^{59}Fe in the rat, *Blood,* 43, 693, 1974.

63. **Jeffcoat, M. K., McNeil, B. J., and Davis, M. A.,** Indium and iron as tracers for erythroid precursors, *J. Nucl. Med.,* 19, 496, 1978.

64. **Harris, W. R.,** Thermodynamic binding constants of the zinc-human serum transferrin complex, *Biochemistry,* 22, 3920, 1983.

65. **Durbin, P. W.,** Plutonium in man: a new look at the old data, in *Radiobiology of Plutonium,* Stover, B. J. and Jee, W. S. S., Eds., John Wiley & Sons, Salt Lake City, 1972, 469.

66. **Stover, B. J., Bruenger, F. W., and Stevens, W.,** The reaction of Pu(IV) with the iron transport system in human blood serum, *Radiat. Res.,* 33, 381, 1968.

67. **Chen, D. C. P., Newman, B., Turkall, R. M., and Tsan, M. F.,** Transferrin receptors and gallium-67 uptake *in vitro, Eur. J. Nucl. Med.,* 7, 536, 1982.

68. **Larson, S. M., Rasey, J. S., Nelson, N. J., Grunbaum, Z., Allen, D. R., Hapr, G. D., and Williams, D. L.,** The kinetics of uptake and macromolecular binding of Ga-67 and Fe-59 by the EMT-6 sarcoma-like tumor of balb/c mice, *Radiopharmaceuticals,* 2, 297, 1979.

69. **Sephton, R. G., De Abrew, S., and Hodgson, G. S.,** Mechanisms of distribution of gallium 67 in mouse tumour hosts, *Br. J. Radiol.,* 55, 134, 1982.

70. **Vallabhajosula, S. R., Harwig, J. F., and Siemsen, J. K.,** Radiogallium localization in tumors: blood binding and transport and the role of transferrin, *Nucl. Med.,* 21, 650, 1980.

71. **Zweier, J., Aiscn, P., Pelsach, J., and Mims, W. B.,** Pulsed electroparamagnetic resonance studies of the copper complexes of transferrin, *J. Biol. Chem.,* 254, 3512, 1978.

72. **Morgan, E. H., Huebers, H., and Finch, C. A.,** Differences between the binding sites for iron binding and release in human and rat transferrin, *Blood,* 52, 1219, 1978.

73. **Morgan, E. H.,** Effect of pH and iron content of transferrin on its binding to reticulocyte receptors, *Biochim. Biophys. Acta,* 762, 498, 1983.

74. **Zapolski, E. J., Ganz, R., and Princiotto, J. V.,** Biological specificity of the iron-binding sites of transferrin, *Am. J. Physiol.,* 226, 334, 1974.

75. **Graham, I. and Williams, J.,** A comparison of glycopeptides from the transferrins of several species, *Biochem. J.,* 145, 263, 1975.

76. **Fransson, G. B., Thoren-Tolling, K., Jones, B., et al.,** Absorption of lactoferrin-iron in suckling pigs, *Nutr. Res.,* 3, 373, 1983.

77. **Spik, G., Bayard, B., Fournet, B., Stecker, G., Bouquelet, S., and Montreuil, J.,** Studies on glycoconjugates. LXIV. Complete structure of two carbohydrate units of human serotransferrin, *FEBS Lett.,* 50, 296, 1975.

78. **Thibodeau, S. N., Lee, D. C., and Palmiter, R. D.,** Identical precursors for serum transferrin and egg white conalbumin, *J. Biol. Chem.,* 252, 3771, 1978.

79. **Bloch, B., Popovici, T., Levin, M. J., Tuil, D., and Kahn, A.,** Transferrin gene expression visualized in oligodendrocytes of the rat brain by using *in situ* hybridization and immunohistochemistry, *Proc. Natl. Acad. Sci. U.S.A.,* 82, 6706, 1985.

80. **Gallo, P., Bracco, F., Morara, S., Battistin, L., and Tavolato, B.,** The cerebrospinal fluid transferrin tau proteins, *J. Neurol. Sci.,* 70, 81, 1985.

81. **Morgan, E. H., Marsaglia, G., Giblett, E. R., and Finch, C. A.,** A method of investigating internal iron exchange utilizing two types of transferrin, *J. Lab Clin. Med.,* 69, 370, 1967.

82. **Dekker, C. J., Kroos, M. J., Van der Heul, C., and Van Eijk, H. G.,** Uptake of sialo and asialo transferrins by isolated rat hepatocytes. Comparison for a heterologous and a homologous system, *Int. J. Biochem.,* 17, 701, 1985.

83. **Bocci, V.,** The role of sialic acid in determining the life span of circulating cells and glycoproteins, *Experientia,* 32, 135, 1976.

84. **Regoeczi, E. and Hatton, M. W. C.,** Transferrin catabolism in mammalian species of different body sizes, *Am. J. Physiol.,* 238, 306, 1980.

85. **Hatton, M. W. C., Marz, L., Berry, L. R., et al.,** Bi- and tri-antennary human transferrin glycopeptides and their affinities for the hepatic lectin specific for asialo-glycoproteins, *Biochem. J.,* 181, 633, 1979.

86. **Regoeczi, E., Chindemi, P. A., and Debanne, M. T.,** Partial resialylation of human asialotransferrin types 1 and 2 in the rat, *Can. J. Biochem. Cell Biol.,* 62, 853, 1984.

87. **Regoeczi, E., Chindemi, P. A., Devanne, M. T., et al.,** Partial resialylation of human asialotransferrin type 3 in the rat, *Proc. Natl. Acad. Sci. U.S.A.,* 79, 2226, 1982.

88. **Stibler, H., Sydow, O., and Berg, S.,** Quantitative estimation of abnormal microheterogeneity of serum transferrin in alcoholics, *Pharmacol. Biochem. Behav.,* 1, 14, 1980.

89. **Van Eijk, H. G., Van Noort, W. L., and Van der Heul, C.,** Microheterogeneity of human serum transferrins: a consequence for immunochemical determinations?, *Clin. Chim. Acta,* 126, 193, 1982.

90. **Rosseneu-Moutreff, M. Y., Soetewey, F., Lamote, R., and Peeters, H.,** Size and shape determination of apotransferrin and transferrin monomers, *Biopolymers,* 10, 1039, 1971.

91. **Martel, P., Kim, S. M., and Powell, B. M.,** Physical characteristics of human transferrin from small angle neutron scattering, *Biophys. J.,* 31, 371, 1980.

92. **Jarritt, P. H.,** Effect of iron on sedimentation-velocity and gel filtration behavior of transferrins from several vertebrates, *Biochim. Biophys. Acta,* 453, 332, 1976.

93. **Palmour, R. M. and Sutton, H. E.,** Vertebrate transferrins. Molecular weights, chemical composition, and iron-binding studies, *Biochemistry,* 10, 4026, 1971.

94. **Yeh, Y., Iwai, S., and Feeney, R. E.,** Conformations of denatured and renatured ovotransferrin, *Biochemistry,* 18, 882, 1979.

95. **Putnam, F. W.,** Transferrin, in *The Plasma Proteins,* 2nd ed., Putnam, F. W., Ed., Academic Press, New York, 1975, 265.

96. **Goodfellow, P., Banting, G., Sutherland, R., Greaves, M., Solomon, E., and Povey, S.,** Expression of human transferrin receptor is controlled by a gene on chromosome 3: assignment using species specificity of a monoclonal antibody, *Som. Cell. Genet.,* 8, 197, 1982.

97. **Enns, C. A., Suomalaninen, H., Gebhardt, J., Schroder, J., and Sussman, H. H.,** Human transferrin receptor: expression of the receptor is assigned to chromosome 3, *Proc. Natl. Acad. Sci. U.S.A.,* 79, 3241, 1982.

98. **Miller, Y. E., Jones, C., Scoggin, C., et al.,** Chromosome 3q (22-ter) encodes the human transferrin receptor, *Am. J. Hum. Genet.,* 33, 573, 1983.

99. **van de Rijn, M., van Kessel, A. H. M. G., Kroezen, V., et al.,** Localization of a gene controlling the expression of the human transferrin receptor to the region q12-qter of chromosome 3, *Cytogenet. Cell Genet.,* 36, 25, 1983.

100. **Sparkes, R. S., Field, L. L., Sparkes, M. C., et al.,** Genetic linkage studies of transferrin, pseudocholinesterase and chromosome 1 loci, *Hum. Hered.,* 34, 96, 1984.

101. **Chibani, J., Lefranc, G., and Constans, J.,** Serum protein polymorphism among Tunisian Berbers: haptoglobin, transferrin and group-specific component subtypes, C3 and BF types, *Ann. Hum. Biol.,* 12, 449, 1985.

102. **Sebetan, I. M., Hiraiwa, K., and Akaishi, S.,** Genetic polymorphism of transferrin in Egyptians: analysis by two electro-focusing methods with description of unusual B variant, *Jpn. J. Hum. Genet.,* 30, 15, 1985.

103. **Matsuda, R., Spector, D., Micou-Eastwood, J., et al.,** There is selective accumulation of a growth factor in chicken skeletal muscle, *Dev. Biol.,* 103, 276, 1984.

104. **Stratil, A., Bobak, P., Tomasek, V., et al.,** Transferrins of barbus, barbus meridionalis petenyi and their hybrids. Genetic polymorphism, heterogeneity and partial characterization, *Comp. Biochem. Physiol.,* 76B, 845, 1983.

105. **Kueppers, F. and Harpel, B. M.,** Transferrin C subtypes in US blacks and whites, *Hum. Hered.,* 30, 376, 1980.

106. **Turnbull, A. and Giblett, E. R.,** The binding and transport of iron by transferrin variants, *J. Lab. Clin. Med.,* 57, 450, 1961.

107. **Evans, R. W., Williams, J., and Moreton, K.,** A variant of human transferrin with abnormal properties, *Biochem. J.,* 201, 19, 1982.

108. **Alper, C. A., Raum, D., Awdeh, Z. L., et al.,** Studies of hepatic synthesis *in vivo* of plasma proteins, including orosomucoid, transferrin, antitrypsin, C8 and factor B1, *Clin. Immunol. Immunopathol.,* 16, 84, 1974.

109. **McKnight, G. S., Lee, D. C., Hemmaplardh, D., et al.,** Transferrin gene expression, *J. Biol. Chem.,* 255, 144, 1980.

110. **McKnight, G. S., Lee, D. C., and Palmiter, R. D.,** Transferrin gene expression, *J. Biol. Chem.,* 255, 148, 1980.

111. **Morton, A. G. and Tavill, A. S.,** The role of iron in the regulation of hepatic transferrin synthesis, *Br. J. Haematol.,* 36, 383, 1977.

112. **Vassy, J., Rissel, M., Kraemer, M., Foucrier, J., et al.,** Ultrastructural indirect immunolocalization of transferrin in cultured rat hepatocytes permeabilized with saponin, *J. Histochem. Cytochem.*, 32, 538, 1984.

113. **Lane, R. S.,** Changes in plasma transferrin levels following the administration of iron, *Br. J. Haematol.*, 12, 249, 1966.

114. **Jeejeebhoy, K. N., Ho, J., Greenberg, G. R., et al.,** Albumin, fibrinogen and transferrin synthesis in isolated rat hepatocyte suspensions, *Biochem. J.*, 146, 141, 1975.

115. **Plant, P. W., Deeley, R. G., and Grieninger, G.,** Selective block of albumin gene expression in chick embryo hepatocytes cultured without hormones and its partial reversal by insulin, *J. Biol. Chem.*, 258, 15355, 1983.

116. **Schreiber, G., Dryburgh, H., Millership, A., et al.,** The synthesis and secretion of rat transferrin, *J. Biol. Chem.*, 254, 12013, 1979.

117. **Morgan, E. H. and Peters, T.,** The biosynthesis of rat serum albumin. V. Effect of protein depletion and refeeding on albumin and transferrin synthesis, *J. Biol. Chem.*, 246, 3500, 1971.

118. **Hochwald, G. M., Jacobson, E. B., and Thorbecke, G. J.,** ^{14}C-amino acid incorporation into transferrin and B24-globulin by ectodesual glands *in vitro*, *Fed. Proc.*, 23, 557, 1964.

119. **Jordan, S. M. and Morgan, E. H.,** Plasma protein synthesis by tissue slices from pregnant and lactating rats, *Biochim. Biophys. Acta*, 174, 373, 1969.

120. **Dickson, P. W., Aldred, A. R., Marley, P. D., Guo-Fen, T., Howlett, G. J., and Schreiber, G.,** High prealbumin and transferrin mRNA levels in the choroid plexus of rat brain, *Biochim. Biophys. Res. Commun.*, 127, 890, 1985.

121. **Prunier, J. H., Bearn, A. G., and Cleve, H.,** Site of formation of the group-specific component and certain other serum protein, *Proc. Soc. Exp. Biol. Med.*, 115, 1005, 1964.

122. **Soltys, H. D. and Brody, J. I.,** Synthesis of transferrin by human peripheral blood lymphocytes, *J. Lab. Clin. Med.*, 75, 250, 1970.

123. **Haurani, F. I., Meyer, A., and O'Brien, R.,** Production of transferrin by the macrophage, *J. Immunol.*, 99, 660, 1967.

124. **Stecher, V. J. and Thorbecke, G. J.,** Sites of synthesis of serum proteins, *J. Immunol.*, 99, 660, 1967.

125. **Asofsky, R. and Thorbecke, G. J.,** Sites of formation of immune globulins and of a component of C'3. II. Production of immunoelectrophoretically identified serum proteins by human and monkey tissues *in vitro*, *J. Exp. Med.*, 14, 471, 1961.

126. **Phillips, M. E. and Thorbecke, G. J.,** Studies on the serum proteins of chimeras. I. Identification and study of the site of origin of Doner type serum protein in adult rat into mouse chimeras, *Int. Arch. Allergy Appl. Immunol.*, 29, 553, 1966.

127. **Morell, A. G., Gregoriadis, G., and Scheinberg, I. H.,** The role of sialic acid in determining the survival of glycoproteins in the circulation, *J. Biol. Chem.*, 246, 1461, 1971.

128. **Jandl, J. H. and Katz, J. H.,** The plasma-to-cell cycle of transferrin, *J. Clin. Invest.*, 42, 314, 1963.

129. **Booth, A. G. and Wilson, M. J.,** Human placental coated vesicles contain receptor-bound transferrin, *Biochem. J.*, 196, 355, 1981.

130. **Ecarot-charrier, B., Grey, V. L., Wilczynska, A., et al.,** Reticulocyte membrane transferrin receptors, *Can. J. Biochem.*, 58, 418, 1980.

131. **Enns, C. A. and Sussman, H. H.,** Physical characterization of the transferrin receptor in human placentae, *J. Biol. Chem.*, 255, 9820, 1981.

132. **Seligman, P. A., Schleicher, R. B., and Allen, R. H.,** Isolation and characterization of the transferrin receptors from human placenta, *J. Biol. Chem.*, 254, 9943, 1979.

133. **VanBockxmeer, F. M. and Morgan, E. H.,** Identification of transferrin receptors in reticulocytes, *Biochim. Biophys. Acta*, 468, 437, 1977.

134. **Verhoef, N. J. and Noordeloos, P. J.,** Binding of transferrin and uptake of iron by rat erythroid cells *in vitro*, *Clin Sci. Mol. Med.*, 52, 87, 1977.

135. **Light, N. D.,** The isolation and partial characterization of transferrin binding components of the rabbit reticulocyte plasma membrane, *Biochim. Biophys. Acta*, 495, 46, 1977.

136. **Light, N. D. and Tanner, M. J. A.,** Changes in surface-membrane components during the differentiation of rabbit erythroid cells, *Biochem. J.*, 164, 565, 1977.

137. **Witt, D. P. and Woodworth, R. C.,** Identification of the transferin receptor of the rabbit reticulocyte, *Biochemistry*, 17, 391, 1978.

138. **Trowbridge, I. S. and Omary, M. B.,** Human cell surface glycoprotein related to cell proliferation is the receptor for transferrin, *Proc. Natl. Acad. Sci. U.S.A.*, 78, 3039, 1981.

139. **Goding, J. W. and Burns, G. F.,** Monoclonal antibody OKT-9 recognizes the receptor for transferrin on human acute lymphocytic leukemia cells, *J. Immunol.*, 127, 1256, 1981.

140. **Sutherland, R., Delia, D., Schneider, C., et al.,** Ubiquitous cell-surface glycoprotein on tumor cells is proliferation-associated receptor for transferrin, *Proc. Natl. Acad. Sci. U.S.A.*, 78, 4515, 1980.

141. **Glass, J., Nunez, M. T., and Robinson, S. H.,** Transferrin-binding and iron-binding proteins of rabbit reticulocyte plasma membranes three distinct moieties, *Biochim. Biophys. Acta*, 598, 293, 1980.

142. **Iacopetta, B. J., Morgan, E. H., and Yeoh, G. C. T.,** Transferrin receptors and iron uptake during erythroid cell development, *Biochim. Biophys. Acta*, 687, 204, 1982.
143. **Steiner, M.,** Fluorescence microphotometric studies of the transferrin receptor in human erythroid precursor cells, *J. Lab. Clin. Med.*, 96, 1086, 1980.
145. **Iacopetta, B. J., Morgan, E. H., and Yeoh, G. C. T.,** Receptor-mediated endocytosis of transferrin by developing erythroid cells from the fetal rat liver, *J. Histochem. Cytochem.*, 31, 336, 1983.
146. **Wada, H. G., Hass, P. E., and Sussman, H. H.,** Transferrin receptor in human placental brush-border membranes, *J. Biol. Chem.*, 254, 12629, 1979.
147. **Hamilton, T. A., Wada, H. G., and Sussman, H. H.,** Identification of transferrin receptors on the surface of human cultured cells, *Proc. Natl. Acad. Sci. U.S.A.*, 76, 6406, 1979.
148. **Trowbridge, I. S., Newman, R. A., Domingo, D. L., et al.,** Transferrin receptors: structure and function, *Biochem. Pharmacol.*, 33, 925, 1984.
149. **Schneider, C., Sutherland, R., Newman, R., et al.,** Structural features of the cell surface receptor for transferrin that is recognized, *J. Biol. Chem.*, 257, 8516, 1982.
150. **Omary, M. B. and Trowbridge, I. S.,** Covalent binding of fatty acid to the transferrin receptor in cultured human cells, *J. Biol. Chem.*, 256, 4715, 1981.
151. **Schneider, C., Kurkinen, M., and Greaves, M.,** Isolation of cDNA clones for the human transferrin receptor, *EMBO J.*, 2, 2259, 1983.
152. **Dautry-varsat, A. and Lodish, H. F.,** How receptors bring proteins and particles into cells, *Sci. Am.*, 250, 52, 1984.
153. **Enns, C. A. and Sussman, H. H.,** Similarities between the transferrin receptor proteins on human reticulocytes and human placentae, *J. Biol. Chem.*, 256, 12650, 1981.
154. **Van Agthoven, A., Goridis, C., Naquet, P., et al.,** Structural characteristics of the mouse transferrin receptor, *Eur. J. Biochem.*, 140, 433, 1984.
155. **Nikinmaa, B., Enns, C. A., Tonik, S. E., et al.,** Monoclonal antibodies to a purified human transferrin receptor, *Scand. J. Immunol.*, 20, 441, 1984.
156. **Huebers, H., Csiba, E., Huebers, E., and Finch, C. A.,** Competitive advantage of diferric transferrin in delivering iron to reticulocytes: a comparative study, *Proc. Natl. Acad. Sci. U.S.A.*, 80, 300, 1983.
157. **Huebers, H., Csiba, E., Huebers, E., and Finch, C. A.,** Molecular advantage of diferric transferrin in delivering iron to reticulocytes: a comparative study, *Proc. Soc. Exp. Biol. Med.*, 179, 222, 1985.
158. **Huebers, H., Csiba, E., Josephson, B., Huebers, E., and Finch, C. A.,** Interaction of human diferric transferrin with reticulocytes, *Proc. Natl. Acad. Sci. U.S.A.*, 78, 621, 1982.
159. **Klausner, R. D., Ashwell, G., Van Renswoude, J., Harford, J. B., and Bridges, K. R.,** Binding of apotransferrin to K562 cells: explanation of the transferrin cycle, *Proc. Natl. Acad. Sci. U.S.A.*, 80, 2263, 1983.
160. **Dautry-Varsat, A., Ciechanover, A., and Lodish, H. F.,** pH and the recycling of transferrin during receptor-mediated endocytosis, *Proc. Natl. Acad. Sci. U.S.A.*, 80, 2258, 1983.
161. **Ward, J. H., Kushner, J. P., and Kaplan, J.,** Preference of transferrin receptors for diferric transferrin, in *Structure and Function of Iron Storage and Transport Proteins*, Urushizaki, I., Aisen, P., Listowsky, I., and Drysdale, J. W., Eds., Elsevier, Amsterdam, 1983, 341.
162. **Adam, M., Rodriguez, A., Turbide, C., et al.,** *In vitro* acylation of the transferrin receptor, *J. Biol. Chem.*, 259, 15460, 1984.
163. **Ward, J. H., Jordan, I., Kushner, J. P., et al.,** Heme regulation of HeLa cell transferrin receptor number, *J. Biol. Chem.*, 259, 13235, 1984.
164. **Harding, C., Heuser, J., and Stahl, P.,** Endocytosis and intracellular processing of transferrin and colloidal gold-transferrin in rat reticulocytes: demonstration of a pathway for receptor shedding, *Eur. J. Cell Biol.*, 35, 256, 1984.
165. **Johnstone, R. M., Adam, M., and Pan, B. T.,** The fate of the transferrin receptor during maturation of sheep reticulocytes *in vitro*, *Can. J. Biochem. Cell Biol.*, 62, 1246, 1984.
166. **Jarnum, S. and Lassen, N. A.,** Albumin and transferrin metabolism in infectious and toxic diseases, *Scan. J. Clin. Lab. Invest.*, 13, 357, 1961.
167. **Jensen, H., Bro-Jorgensen, K., Jarnum, S., et al.,** Transferrin metabolism in the nephrotic syndrome and in protein-losing gastroenteropathy, *Scand. J. Clin. Lab. Invest.*, 21, 293, 1968.
168. **Katz, J. H.,** Iron and protein kinetics studied by means of a doubly-labelled human crystalline transferrin, *J. Clin. Invest.*, 40, 2143, 1961.
169. **Masuya, T. and Kozuru, M.,** Clinical and experimental studies on the metabolism of transferrin II. Turnover studies with iodine-labelled human transferrin, *Kyushu J. Med. Sci.*, 14, 233, 1963.
170. **Van der Heul, C., Veldman, A., Kroos, M. J., et al.,** Two mechanisms are involved in the process of iron-uptake by rat reticulocytes, *Int. J. Bichem.*, 16, 383, 1984.
171. **Woodworth, R. C., Brown-Mason, A., Cristensen, T. G., et al.,** An alternative model for the binding and release of diferric transferrin by reticulocytes, *Biochemistry*, 21, 4220, 1982.

172. **Morley, C. G. D. and Bezkorovainy, A.,** Cellular iron uptake from transferrin: is endocytosis the only mechanism?, *Int. J. Biochem.,* 17, 553, 1985.

173. **Iacopetta, B. J. and Morgan, E. H.,** The kinetics of transferrin endocytosis and iron uptake from transferrin in rabbit reticulocytes, *J. Biol. Chem.,* 258, 9108, 1983.

174. **Iacopetta, B. J. and Morgan, E. H.,** An electron-microscope autoradiographic study of transferrin endocytosis by immature erythroid cells, *Eur. J. Cell Biol.,* 32, 17, 1983.

175. **Karin, M. and Mintz, B.,** Receptor-mediated endocytosis of transferrin in developmentally totipotent mouse teratocarcinoma stem cells, *J. Biol. Chem.,* 256, 3245, 1981.

176. **Klausner, R. D., Harford, J., and van Renswoude, J.,** Rapid internalization of the transferrin receptor in K562 cells is triggered by ligand binding or treatment with a phorbol ester, *Proc. Natl. Acad. Sci. U.S.A.,* 81, 3005, 1984.

177. **Klausner, R. D., van Renswoude, J., and Ashwell, G., et al.,** Receptor-mediated endocytosis of transferrin in K562 cells, *J. Biol. Chem.,* 258, 4715, 1983.

178. **Faulk, W. P., Hsi, B. L., and Stevens, P. J.,** Transferrin and transferrin receptors in carcinoma of the breast, *Lancet,* 2, 390, 1980.

179. **Bessis, M. and Breton-Gorius, J.,** Etude au microscope electronique des granulations ferrugineuses des erythrocytes normaux et pathologiques, *Rev. Hematol.,* 12, 43, 1957.

180. **Mattia, E., Rao, K., Shapiro, D. S., et al.,** Biosynthetic regulation of the human transferrin receptor by desferrioxamine in K562 cells, *J. Biol. Chem.,* 259, 2689, 1984.

181. **Larrick, J. W., Enns, C., Raubitschek, A., and Weintraub, H.,** Receptor-mediated endocytosis of human transferrin and its cell surface receptor, *J. Cell. Physiol.,* 124, 183, 1985.

182. **Bomford, A., Young, S. P., and Williams, R.,** Release of iron from the two iron-binding sites of transferrin by cultured human cells: modulation by methylamine, *Biochemistry,* 24, 3472, 1985.

183. **Patterson, S., Armstrong, N. J., Iacopetta, B. J., et al.,** Intravesicular pH and iron uptake by immature erythroid cells, *J. Cell Physiol.,* 120, 225, 1984.

184. **Veldman, A., Kroos, M. J., Van der Heul, C., et al.,** Are lysosomes directly involved in the iron uptake by reticulocytes?, *Int. J. Biochem.,* 16, 39, 1984.

185. **Veldman, A., Van der Heul, C., Kroos, M. J., and VanEijk, H. G.,** Fluorescence probe measurement of the pH of the transferrin microenvironment during iron uptake by rat bone marrow erythroid cells, *Br. J. Haematol.,* 62, 155, 1986.

186. **Egyed, A.,** Studies on the partition of transferrin-donated iron in rabbit reticulocytes. I. The kinetics of iron distribution between stroma and cytosol, *Br. J. Haematol.,* 52, 457, 1982.

187. **Konopka, K. and Romslo, I.,** Studies on the mechanism of pyrophosphate-mediated uptake of iron from transferrin by isolated rat-liver mitochondria, *Eur. J. Biochem.,* 117, 239, 1981.

188. **Dickson, R. B., Hanover, J. A., Willingham, M. C., et al.,** Prelysosomal divergence of transferrin and epidermal growth factor during receptor-mediated endocytosis, *Biochemistry,* 22, 5667, 1983.

189. **Tso, S. C., Loh, T. T., and Todd, D.,** Iron overload in patients with haemoglobin H disease, *Scand. J. Haematol.,* 32, 391, 1981.

190. **Stein, B. S., Bensch, K. G., and Sussman, H. H.,** Complete inhibition of transferrin recycling by monensin in K562 cells, *J. Biol. Chem.,* 259, 14762, 1984.

191. **Hebbert, D. and Morgan, E. H.,** Calmodulin antagonists inhibit and phorbol esters enhance transferrin endocytosis and iron uptake by immature erythroid cells, *Blood,* 65, 758, 1985.

192. **Hemmaplardh, D. and Morgan, E. H.,** The role of calcium in transferrin and iron uptake by reticulocytes, *Biochim. Biophys. Acta,* 468, 423, 1977.

193. **Nunez, M. T. and Glass, J.,** Reconstitution of the transferrin receptor in lipid vesicles. Effect of cholesterol on the binding of transferrin, *Biochemistry,* 21, 4139, 1982.

194. **Chaudhuri, T. K., Ehrhardt, J. C., and DeGowin, R. L., et al.,** 59Fe whole-body scanning, *J. Nucl. Med.,* 15, 667, 1974.

195. **Muller, C. P., Volloch, Z., and Shinitzky, M.,** Correlation between cell density, membrane fluidity, and the availability of transferrin receptors in Friend erythroleukemic cells, *Cell Biophys.,* 2, 233, 1980.

196. **Wiley, H. S. and Kaplan, J.,** Epidermal growth factor rapidly induces a redistribution of transferrin receptor pools in human fibroblasts, *Proc. Natl. Acad. Sci. U.S.A.,* 81, 7456, 1984.

197. **Kontoghiorghes, G. J. and Evans, R. W.,** Site specificity of iron removal from transferrin by α-keto-hydroxypyridine chelators, *FEBS Lett.,* 189, 141, 1985.

198. **Fletcher, J.,** Variation in the availability of transferrin-bound iron for uptake by immature red cells, *Clin. Sci. Mol. Med.,* 37, 273, 1969.

199. **Fletcher, J. and Huehns, E. R.,** Function of transferrin, *Nature,* 218, 1211, 1968.

200. **Zapolski, E. J. and Princiottto, J. V.,** Preferential utilization *in vitro* of iron bound to diferric transferrin by rabbit reticulocytes, *Biochem. J.,* 166, 175, 1977.

201. **Awai, M., Chipman, B., and Brown, E. B.,** *In vivo* evidence for the functional heterogeneity of transferrin-bound iron. II. Studies in pregnant rats, *J. Lab. Clin. Med.,* 85, 785, 1975.

202. **Hahn, D.,** Functional behaviour of transferrin, *J. Biochem.,* 34, 311, 1973.

203. **Hahn, D., Baviera, B., and Ganzoni, A. M.,** Functional heterogeneity of the transport iron compartment, *Acta Haematol.,* 53, 285, 1975.

204. **van Baarlen, J., Brouwer, J. T., Leibman, A., and Aisen, P.,** Evidence for the functional heterogeneity of the two sites of transferrin *in vitro, Br. J. Haematol.,* 46, 417, 1981.

205. **Verhoef, N. J., Kottenhagen, M. J., Mulder, H. J. M., et al.,** Functional heterogeneity of transferrin-bound iron, *Acta Haematol.,* 60, 210, 1978.

206. **Kim, B. K., Huebers, H. A., Pippard, M. J., and Finch, C. A.,** Storage iron exchange in the rat as affected by deferrioxamine, *J. Lab. Clin. Med.,* 105, 440, 1985.

207. **Garrett, N. E., Garrett, R. J. B., and Archdeacon, J. W.,** Solubilization and chromatography of iron-binding compounds from reticulocyte stroma, *Biochem. Biophys. Res. Commun.,* 52, 446, 1973.

208. **Mitchell, J., Halden, E. R., Jones, F., et al.,** Lowering of transferrin during iron absorption in iron deficiency, *J. Lab. Clin. Med.,* 56, 555, 1960.

209. **Makey, D. G. and Seal, U. S.,** The detection of four molecular forms of human transferrin during the iron binding process, *Biochim. Biophys. Acta,* 453, 250, 1976.

210. **Leibman, A. and Aisen, P.,** Distribution of iron between the binding sites of transferrin serum: methods and results in normal human subjects, *Blood,* 43, 1058, 1979.

211. **Huebers, H. A., Josephson, B., Huebers, E., Csiba, E., and Finch, C. A.,** Occupancy of the iron binding sites of human transferrin, *Proc. Natl. Acad. Sci. U.S.A.,* 81, 4326, 1984.

212. **DiRusso, S. C., Check, I. J., and Hunter, R. L.,** Quantitation of apo-, mono-, and diferric transferrin by polyacrylamide gradient gel electrophoresis in patients with disorders of iron metabolism, *Blood,* 66, 1445, 1985.

213. **Huebers, H., Josephson, B., Huebers, E., Csiba, E., and Finch, C. A.,** Uptake and release of iron from human transferrin, *Proc. Natl. Acad. Sci. U.S.A.,* 78, 2572, 1981.

214. **Delaney, T. A., Morgan, W. H., and Morgan, E. H.,** Chemical, but not functional, differences between the iron-binding sites of rabbit transferrin, *Biochim. Biophys. Acta,* 701, 295, 1982.

215. **Huebers, H., Bauer, W., Huebers, E., Csiba, E., and Finch, C. A.,** The behavior of transferrin iron in the rat, *Blood,* 57, 218, 1981.

216. **Huebers, H., Huebers, E., Csiba, E., and Finch, C. A.,** Iron uptake from rat plasma transferrin by rat reticulocytes, *J. Clin. Invest.,* 62, 1944, 1978.

217. **Van der Huel, C., Kroos, M. J., Van Noort, W. L., et al.,** No functional difference of the two iron-binding sites of human transferrin *in vitro, Clin. Sci.,* 60, 185, 1981.

218. **Van der Heul, C., Kroos, M. J., Van Noort, W. L., et al.,** In vitro and *in vivo* studies of iron delivery by human monoferric transferrins, *Br. J. Haematol.,* 56, 571, 1984.

219. **Van Eijk, H. G., Van Noort, W. L., Kroos, M. J., et al.,** The heterogeneity of human serum transferrin and human transferrin preparations on isolectric focusing gels: no functional difference of the fractions *in vitro, Clin. Chim. Acta,* 121, 209, 1982.

220. **Young, S. P., Bomford, A., and Williams, R.,** The effect of the iron saturation of transferrin on its binding and uptake by rabbit reticulocytes, *Biochem. J.,* 219, 505, 1984.

221. **Heaphy, S. and Williams, J.,** Removal of iron from diferric rabbit serum transferrin by rabbit reticulocytes, *Biochem. J.,* 205, 619, 1982.

222. **Huebers, H., Huebers, E., Csiba, E., and Finch, C. A.,** Heterogeneity of the plasma iron pool: the explanation of the Fletcher-Huehns phenomenon, *Am. J. Physiol.,* 247, R280, 1984.

223. **Testa, U., Titeux, M., Louache, F., et al.,** Transferrin is not an obligatory growth factor for human erythroleukemic cell lines, *Blood,* 62, 127a, 1983.

224. **Lim, B. C. and Morgan, E. H.,** Transferrin-receptor interaction and its significance to protein evolution, 7th Int. Conf. Protein Iron Metab.

225. **Esparza, I. and Brock, J. H.,** The effect of trypsin digestion on the structure and iron-donating properties of transferrins from several species, *Biochim. Biophys. Acta,* 622, 297, 1980.

226. **Bothwell, T. H., Conrad, M. E., Cook, J. D., et al.,** Proposed recommendations for measurement of serum iron in human blood, *Blood,* 37, 598, 1971.

227. **Bothwell, T. H., Pirzio-Biroli, G., and Finch, C. A.,** Iron absorption I. Factors influencing absorption, *J. Lab. Clin. Med.,* 51, 24, 1958.

228. **Hallberg, L.,** Bioavailability of dietary iron in man, *Annu. Rev. Nutr.,* 1, 123, 1981.

229. **Hallberg, L. and Bjorn-Rasmussen, E.,** Determination of iron absorption from whole diet. A new two-pool model using two radioiron isotopes given as haem and non-haem iron, *Scand. J. Haematol.,* 9, 193, 1972.

230. **Heinrich, H. C., Gabbe, E. E., and Kugler, G.,** Comparative absorption of ferri-haemoglobin-59Fe/ferro-haemoglobin-59Fe and $59Fe^{3+}/59Fe^{2+}$ in humans with normal and depleted iron stores, *Eur. J. Clin. Invest.,* 1, 321, 1971.

231. **Muir, A. and Hopfer, U.,** Regional specificity of iron uptake by small intestinal brush-border membranes from normal and iron-deficient mice, *Am. J. Physiol.,* 248, G376, 1985.

232. **Parmley, R. T., Barton, J. C., and Conrad, M. E.,** Utlrastructural cytochemical identification of the siderophilic enterocyte, *J. Histochem. Cytochem.,* 32, 724, 1984.

233. **Parmley, R. T., Barton, J. C., Conrad, M. E., and Austin, R. L.,** Ultrastructural cytochemistry of iron absorption, *Am. J. Pathol.,* 93, 707, 1978.

234. **Conrad, M. E. and Crosby, W. H.,** Intestinal mucosal mechanisms controlling iron absorption, *Blood,* 22, 406, 1963.

235. **Forth, W. and Rummel, W.,** Gastrointestinal absorption of heavy metals, in *IEPT-Pharmacology of Intestinal Absorption: Gastrointestinal Absorption of Drugs, Section 39B,* Pergamon Press, Oxford, 1975, 599.

236. **Gubler, C.,** Absorption and metabolism of iron, *Science,* 123, 87, 1956.

237. **Saddi, R. and Schapira, G.,** Iron requirements during growth, in *Iron Deficiency,* Hallberg, L., Harwerth, H. G., and Vannotti, A., Eds., Academic Press, London, 1970, 183.

238. **Josephs, H. W.,** Iron metabolism and the hypochromic anemia of infancy, *Medicine,* 32, 125, 1953.

239. **Jackson, R. L., et al.,** Growth charts, *J. Pediatr.,* 27, 215, 1945.

241. **Green, R., Charlton, R., Seftel, H., Bothwell, T., Mayet, F., Finch, C. A., and Layrisse, M.,** Body iron excretion in man, *Am. J. Med.,* 45, 336, 1968.

242. **Beaton, G. H.,** Epidemiology of iron deficiency, in *Iron in Biochemistry and Medicine,* Worwood, J., Ed., Academic Press, New York, 1974, chap. 13.

243. **Lipschitz, D. A., Cook, J. D., and Finch, C. A.,** A clinical evaluation of serum ferritin as an index of iron stores, *N. Engl. J. Med.,* 290, 1213, 1974.

244. **Dallman, P. R. and Siimes, M. A.,** Iron deficiency in infancy and childhood, *Rep. Int. Nutr. Anemia Consultative Group,* 1213, 1979.

245. **Hosain, F. and Finch, C. A.,** A study of internal distribution of iron in man, *Acta Med. Scand.,* 445, 256, 1966.

246. **Kahn, E., Aubert, B., Parmentier, C. et al.,** Feasibility of a 59Fe ferrokinetic study based on bone-marrow scans, *Eur. J. Nucl. Med.,* 8, 312, 1983.

247. **Finch, C. A., Deubelbeiss, K., Cook, J. D., et al.,** Ferrokinetics in man, *Medicine,* 49, 17, 1970.

248. **Garby, L. and Noyes, W. D.,** Studies on hemoglobin metabolism. II. Pathways of hemoglobin iron metabolism in normal man, *J. Clin. Invest.,* 38, 1484, 1959.

249. **Hershko, C., Cook, J. D., and Finch, C. A.,** Storage iron kinetics. II. The uptake of hemoglobin iron by hepatic parenchymal cells, *J. Lab. Clin. Med.,* 80, 624, 1972.

250. **Cap, J., Lehotska, V., Mayerova, A.,** Kongenitalna atransferinemia U 11 mcsaciieho dietata, *Cesk. Pediatr.,* 23, 1020, 1968.

251. **Goya, N., Miyazaki, S., Kodate, S., and Ushio, B.,** A family of congenital atransferrinemia, *Blood,* 40, 239, 1972.

252. **Heilmeyer, L.,** Die Atransferrinamien, *Acta Haematol.,* 36, 40, 1966.

253. **Heilmeyer, L., Keller, W., and Vivell, O.,** Congenital transferrin deficiency in a seven-year old girl, *Ger. Med. Methods,* 6, 385, 1961.

254. **Sakata, T.,** Atransferrinemia, *J. Ped. Pract.,* 32, 1523, 1969.

255. **Cazzola, M., Huebers, H. A., Sayers, M. H., MacPhail, A. P., Eng, M., and Finch, C. A.,** Transferrin saturation, plasma iron turnover, and transferrin uptake in normal humans, *Blood,* 66, 935, 1985.

256. **Cazzola, M., Pootrakul, P., Huebers, H., Eng, M., and Finch, C. A.,** The adequacy of iron supply for erythropoiesis: *in vivo* observations in man, *Blood,* 935, 1985.

257. **Koerper, M. A. and Dallman, P. R.,** Serum iron concentration and transferrin saturation in the diagnosis of iron deficiency in children: normal developmental changes, *J. Pediatr.,* 91, 870, 1977.

258. Life Sciences Research Office, Assessment of the Iron Nutritional Status of the U.S. Population Based on Data Collected in the Second National Health and Nutrition Examination Survey, 1976-1980, Pilch, S. M. and Senti, F. R., Eds., FASEB Special Publications Office, Bethesda, MD, 1984, 1.

259. **Milman, N. and Cohn, J.,** Serum iron, serum transferrin and transferrin saturation in healthy children without iron deficiency, *J. Pediatr.,* 143, 96, 1984.

260. **Cook, J. D., Hershko, C., and Finch, C. A.,** Storage iron kinetics. I. Measurement of the cellular distribution of 59Fe in rat liver, *J. Lab. Clin. Med.,* 80, 613, 1972.

261. **Fawwaz, R. A., Winchell, H. S., Pollycove, M., and Sargent, T.,** Hepatic iron deposition in humans. I. First-pass hepatic deposition of intestinally absorbed iron in patients with low plasma latent iron-binding capacity, *Blood,* 30, 417, 1967.

262. **Wheby, M. S. and Umpierre, G.,** Effect of transferrin saturation on iron absorption in man, *N. Engl. J. Med.,* 271, 1391, 1964.

263. **Bothwell, T. H., Pribilla, W. F., Mebust, W., and Finch, C. A.,** Iron metabolism in the pregnant rabbit. Iron transport across the placenta, *Am. J. Physiol.,* 193, 615, 1958.

264. **Finch, C. A., Huebers, H. A., Miller, L., Josephson, B., Shepard, T., and Mackler, B.,** Fetal iron balance in the rat, *Am. J. Clin. Nutr.,* 37, 910, 1983.

265. **Sturgeon, P.,** Studies of iron requirements in infants. Influence of supplemental iron during normal pregnancy on mother and infant, *Br. J. Haematol.,* 5, 31, 1959.
266. **Shott, R. J. and Andrews, B. F.,** Iron status of a medical high-risk population at delivery, *Am. J. Dis. Child.,* 124, 369, 1972.
267. **Fenton, V., Cavill, I., and Fisher, J.,** Iron stores in pregnancy, *Br. J. Haematol.,* 37, 145, 1977.
268. **Rios, E., Hunter, R. E., Cook, J. D., Smith, N. J., and Finch, C. A.,** The absorption of iron as supplements in infant cereal and infant formulas, *Pediatrics,* 55, 686, 1975.
269. **Gerritsen, T. H. and Walker, A. R. P.,** The effect of habitually high iron intake on certain blood values in pregnant Bantu women, *J. Clin. Invest.,* 33, 23, 1954.
270. **Morgan, E. H. and Melb, M. B.,** Plasma-iron and haemoglobin levels in pregnancy, *Lancet,* 1, 23, 1961.
271. **Deiss, A.,** Iron metabolism in reticuloendothelial cells, *Semin. Hematol.,* 20, 81, 1983.
272. **Uchida, T., Akitsuki, T., Camera, H., et al.,** Relationship among plasma iron, plasma iron turnover, and reticuloendothelial iron release, *Blood,* 61, 799, 1983.
273. **Hershko, C., Cook, J. D., and Finch, C. A.,** Storage iron kinetics. VI. The effect of inflammation on iron exchange in the rat, *Br. J. Haematol.,* 26, 67, 1974.
274. **Finch, C. A., Huebers, H. A., Cazzola, M., Bergamaschi, G., and Belloti, V.,** Storage iron, in *Ferritins and Isoferritins as Biochemical Markers,* Albertini, A., Ed., Elsevier/North Holland, Amsterdam, 1985, 3.
275. **Finch, S. C. and Finch, C. A.,** Idiopathic hemochromatosis, an iron storage disease, *Medicine,* 34, 381, 1955.
276. **Pippard, M. J., Johnson, D. K., and Finch, C. A.,** A rapid assay for evaluation of iron-chelating agents in rats, *Blood,* 58, 685, 1981.
277. **Finch, C. A. and Huebers, H.,** Perspectives in iron metabolism, *N. Engl. J. Med.,* 1520, 1982.
278. **Powell, L. W. and Halliday, J. W.,** Iron absorption and overload, *Clin. Gastroenterol.,* 3, 707, 1981.
279. **Halliday, J. W. and Powell, L. W.,** Iron overload, *Semin. Hematol.,* 19, 42, 1982.
280. **Weatherall, D. J.,** The iron-loading anemias, in *Development of Iron Chelators for Clinical Use,* Martell, Anderson, and Badman, Eds., Elsevier/North Holland, Amsterdam, 1981, 3.
281. **Brown, E. B.,** Candidate chelating drugs: where do we stand?, in *Development of Iron Chelators for Clinical Use,* Martell, Anderson, and Badman, Eds., Elsevier/North Holland, Amsterdam, 1981, 45.
282. **Jacobs, A.,** Iron chelation therapy for iron loaded patients, *Br. J. Haematol.,* 43, 1, 1979.
283. **Finch, C. A., Pippard, M. J., and Johnson, D. K.,** Iron pools and screens for iron chelators, in *Development of Iron Chelators for Clinical Use,* Martell, Anderson, and Badman, Eds., Elsevier/North Holland, 1981, 33.
284. **Pitt, C. G.,** Structure and activity relationships of iron chelating drugs, in *Development of Iron Chelators for Clinical Use,* Martell, Anderson, and Badman, Eds., Elsevier/North Holland, 1981, 105.
285. **Pitt, C. G., Gupta, G., Estes, W. E., et al.,** The selection and evaluation of new chelating agents for the treatment of iron overload, *J. Pharmacol. Exp. Ther.,* 208, 12, 1979.
286. **Hussain, M. A. M., Flynn, D. M., Green, N., et al.,** Subcutaneous infusion and intramuscular injection of desferrioxamine in patients with transfusional iron overload, *Lancet,* 2, 1278, 1976.
287. **Pippard, M. J., Warner, G. T., Callender, S. T., et al.,** Iron absorption in iron-loading anaemias: effect of subcutaneous desferrioxamine infusions, *Lancet,* 2, 737, 1977.
288. **Propper, R. D., Cooper, B., Rufo, R. R., et al.,** Continuous subcutaneous administration of deferoxamine in patients with iron overload, *N. Engl. J., Med.,* 297, 418, 1977.
289. **Hershko, C. and Rachmilewitz, E. A.,** Mechanism of desferrioxamine-induced iron excretion in thalassaemia, *Br. J. Haematol.,* 42, 125, 1979.
290. **Summers, M. R., Jacobs, A., Tudway, D., et al.,** Studies in desferrioxamine and ferrioxamine metabolism in normal and iron-loaded subjects, *Br. J. Haematol.,* 42, 547, 1979.
291. **Drysdale, J. W. and Munro, H. N.,** Regulation of synthesis and turnover of ferritin in rat liver, *J. Biol. Chem.,* 241, 3630, 1966.
292. **Hershko, C., Grady, R. W., and Link, G.,** Development and evaluation of the improved iron chelating agents EHPG, HBED and their dimethyl esters, *Haematology,* 17, 25, 1984.
293. **Brown, J. P., Hewick, R. M., Hellstrom, I., et al.,** Human melanoma-associated antigen p97 is structurally and functionally related to transferrin, *Nature,* 296, 171, 1982.
294. **Plowman, G. D., Brown, J. P., Enns, C. A., et al.,** Assignment of the gene for the human melanoma-associated antigen p97 to chromosome 3, *Nature,* 303, 70, 1983.
295. **Hillman, R. S. and Finch, C. A.,** *Red Cell Manual,* 5th ed., F. A. Davis, Philadelphia, 1985, 1.
296. **Huebers, H. A.,** Iron overload: pathogenesis and treatment with chelating agents, *Blut,* 47, 61, 1983.
297. **Huebers, H.,** unpublished data.
298. **Bergamaschi, M.,** unpublished data.

Chapter 2

HEMATOPOIESIS AND STORAGE IRON IN INFANTS

Martti A. Siimes

TABLE OF CONTENTS

I. INTRODUCTION

Many clinicians argue whether a healthy woman needs iron supplementation during her pregnancy. There is supporting data both against and for the use of extra iron. Nevertheless, it is clear that there is an elevated need for iron during pregnancy compared to a situation where the same woman would have continued average menstruation without being pregnant. Calculations indicate that average iron reserves are about 200 to 300 mg in an adult woman and that the requirements during pregnancy are approximately 1000 mg. Increased absorption of iron should account for at least part of this difference and usually prevents the appearance of any sign of anemia, at least in societies without nutritional deficiencies. Ishikawa et al. have recently published an interesting study where they followed 32 healthy women through and after pregnancy.[1] No iron supplement was received by 20 of the subjects throughout the study; 12 of the subjects received a large dose of iron (800 mg of elemental iron as iron-chondroitinsulfate colloid) intravenously, starting at the 22nd week of pregnancy. This treatment significantly elevated the hemoglobin concentrations in mid- and late pregnancy. Serum ferritin concentration increased during pregnancy and the rise also continued after pregnancy; however, this dose of iron did not prevent the decrease in serum ferritin concentration during the weeks prior to birth indicating that there is both iron-dependent and iron-independent physiological regulation of serum ferritin concentration in pregnancy. It is far from clear how the iron status of a pregnant woman is reflected in her fetus and subsequently in her infant during lactation.

II. HEMATOPOIESIS

A. HEMATOPOIESIS IN THE FETUS

Several developmental changes occur in the erythropoiesis of the fetus. The site of red blood cell production is primarily in liver tissues by 3 months of gestation age. The bone marrow takes over gradually, starting around 5 months of gestation age (Figure 1). Usually by term of pregnancy, the bone marrow is almost exclusively responsible for erythropoiesis. In preterm newborns, the liver plays a role in red blood cell production even at birth. There are also other developmental changes that occur simultaneously. The size of the red cell gradually becomes smaller during fetal life so that the red cell mean corpuscular volume (MCV) tends to be larger in premature than in full-term newborns. The concentration of hemoglobin seems to rise in the fetus during pregnancy although the details of this development are not well known. Finally, the specific fetal hemoglobin-F is partially replaced by adult hemoglobin-A by term of pregnancy. Thus, premature infants have proportionally more hemoglobin-F than full-term newborns.

B. HEMATOPOIESIS IN LOW-BIRTH-WEIGHT INFANTS

Low-birth-weight infants cannot manage to maintain optimal iron nutrition without iron supplementation after the age of about 2 months. The concentration of hemoglobin and the values for MCV of red blood cells, transferrin iron saturation, and serum ferritin all tend to be significantly lower in the unsupplemented infants after this age.[2] The difference in the concentration of hemoglobin averaged from 1 to 2 g/dl in such conditions during a follow-up period of up to 6 months.[2] This difference would have been greater if many of the unsupplemented infants had not been started on iron medication after the documentation of anemia in this particular study.

General recommendations are required for an optimal quality of iron supplementation even if the individual needs for iron may vary with birth weight, neonatal sickness, and blood loss. In the birth weight category between 1000 and 2000 g, available data indicate that iron-supplemented infants given 2 mg iron per kilogram per day do not show evidence

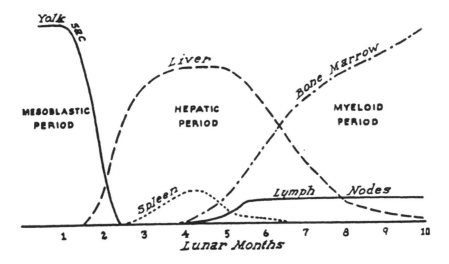

FIGURE 1. Site of fetal erythropoiesis in the developing embryo and fetus.

of clinically significant iron deficiency.[2] This dose, therefore, seems adequate for erythro-poiesis, but is certainly not excessive for the maintenance of a reserve of storage iron. A high frequency of borderline serum ferritin values were found in the supplemented prematures although no anemia was documented.[2] It could be argued that a higher dose of iron, such as 3 mg/kg/day, would provide a more comfortable margin of safety, especially in those infants with birth weight between 1000 and 1500 g.

In another investigation, 62 low-birth-weight infants (birth weight from 850 to 2450 g) were assigned to receive either Fe^{2+} or Fe^{3+}, in different doses (Fe^{2+} 9.6 mg/d or Fe^{3+} 27.5 mg/d elemental iron, respectively). Iron supplementation was started at the age of 6 weeks.[3] No significant differences between the two groups given iron were noted in any of the blood values. Within the Fe^{2+} group, infants demonstrated symptoms, such as colic, excessive crying, constipation, and, in one infant, loose stools. In four infants, both colic and constipation were noted. Fe^{2+} was discontinued in seven infants: two infants with constipation had normal stools after switching to Fe^{3+}, and treatment was discontinued completely in five infants. Among infants given Fe^{3+}, 15% had gastrointestinal problems, and medication was stopped in three (one with colic, one with excessive crying, and one with diarrhea that ceased when the child was given Fe^{2+}). The authors suggest that both Fe^{2+} and Fe^{3+} preparations appear to have a place in the prevention of the late anemia in preterm infants.[3]

Some recent data indicate that use of 4 mg of iron per kilogram per day in a group of very low-birth-weight infants with a birth weight of less than 1000 g prevented most of the chemical and laboratory signs of iron deficiency as demonstrated in Figure 2.[4] Figure 3 illustrates the laboratory data at ages 4, 9, and 15 months. There was a marked decline in serum ferritin despite this large dose of iron during this age period. It is surprising, however, that only a few low values of serum ferritin were found even if iron needs of this infant population were extraordinarily high.

C. MAINTENANCE OF HEMOGLOBIN CONCENTRATION

Preterm infants present a fall in hemoglobin concentration during the first 2 months of life that is more marked than in term infants (Table 1). It also seems that the fall is dependent on the birth weight, even if presumptively adequate iron nutrition is guaranteed (Figure 2). Thus, the early anemia of prematurity, which results in minimum hemoglobin values at age 2 months, cannot be prevented by any known means of iron or vitamin supplementation and therefore it might be considered physiologic.

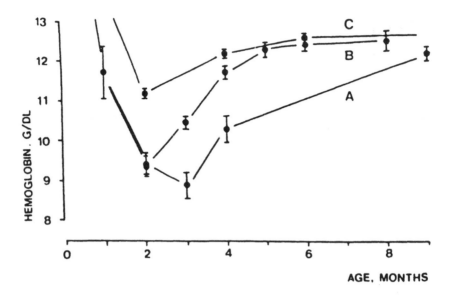

FIGURE 2. Hemoglobin concentration in iron-supplemented infants after birth. A = BW <1000 g, iron dose 4 mg/kg/d, B = BW about 1500 g, iron dose 2 mg/kg/d, C = Full-term infants, iron dose 1 mg/kg/d.

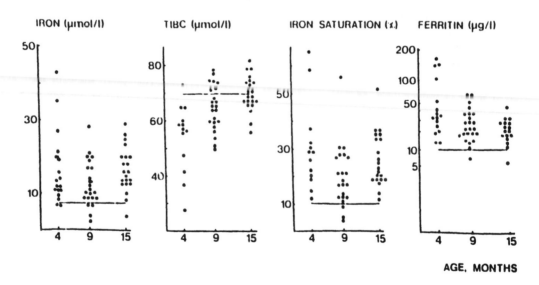

FIGURE 3. Iron status of very low-birth-weight infants up to age 15 months after birth.[4] The infants received about 4 mg iron per kilogram per day. The horizontal lines indicate the limits which might be considered as normal in full-term infants.

It has been demonstrated that in spite of the great demands of rapid growth and the rapid increase of blood volume, low-birth-weight infants with a birth weight above 1000 g attain the level of erythrocyte count, hemoglobin concentration, and red cell indices of term infants during the first half year of life when sufficient iron has been administered.[5] Therefore, prematurity alone cannot be regarded as the cause of red blood cell values that are lower than in normal infants after the age of 6 months.

Very low-birth-weight infants with a birth weight less than 1000 g form an exceptional group among the prematures. The increasing number of surviving very low-birth-weight

TABLE 1
Hemoglobin Concentration in Low-Birth-Weight Infants (Infants were Supplemented with Iron and Vitamins)[2,4]

Age	Birth weight	
	1000—1500 g	1501—2000 g
2 weeks	16.3 (11.7—18.4)	14.8 (11.8—19.6)
1 months	10.9 (8.7—15.2)	11.5 (8.2—15.0)
2 months	8.8 (7.1—11.5)	9.4 (8.0—11.4)
3 months	9.8 (8.9—11.2)	10.2 (9.3—11.8)
4 months	11.3 (9.1—13.1)	11.3 (9.1—13.1)
5 months	11.6 (10.2—14.3)	11.8 (10.4—13.0)
6 months	12.0 (9.4—13.8)	11.8 (10.7—12.6)

infants emphasizes their clinical role although only about or less than 100 such infants are born annually per million of the general population in many developed countries.

Infants with a birth weight of 1000 g or less have a remarkably rapid rate of postnatal growth and unusually high nutritional requirements particularly during their first year of life. In many cases, the birth weight is increased tenfold or more during the subsequent 15 months which is an outstanding figure in man. However, there is an unusually large individual variation in the weight gain and consequently in the iron need. One might anticipate that the concentration of hemoglobin would be the lowest in those infants with most rapid rate of growth. However, there was no significant relationship between these parameters (Figure 4) at any age shown in a group of such infants.[4] Even very low-birth-weight infants are thus apparently capable to accommodate the intestinal absorption of iron needed for their high needs. The lack of a relationship between growth rate and the remarkable catch-up in hemoglobin concentration not only argues against the likelihood that iron is rate-limiting in hemoglobin production under these conditions, but also makes it less likely that a deficiency of other nutrients could play a major role in restricting hemoglobin production during late infancy.

It is interesting that the catch-up of normal hemoglobin concentration seems to take considerably longer time in the prematures with birth weight less than 1000 g than in larger premature infants (Figure 2) although they were supplemented with iron, 4 mg/kg/d and there was little or no evidence of iron deficiency (Figure 3).

It is rare that an infant with a birth weight less than 1000 g is treated without many laboratory studies, yet those who were, were able to compensate remarkably well for the blood loss caused by the sampling.[4] There are some infants reported who required no transfusions and still maintained their subsequent hemoglobin concentrations at a level similar to those infants who were given transfusions (Table 2). This is another indication that regulation of iron absorption is well developed in these very small and rapidly growing infants and that provision of additional iron can effectively prevent the development of iron deficiency. The correlation between iron intake and iron absorption in six preterm infants who received no blood transfusions indicates that the infants exert no control over iron absorption which is a function of the concentration of the diet.[6] Thus, if they are given too much iron they will also absorb too much and if given too little they will absorb insufficiently (Figure 5). The author further estimated that 5 mg of iron per kilogram per day would result in a retention of iron close to that occurring *in utero*, but about 2.5 mg of iron per kilogram per day would probably suffice for the rise in hemoglobin mass.[6]

The fall in hemoglobin concentration of low-birth-weight infants is associated with a relatively rapid fall in MCV of red blood cells which is more rapid than that found in full-term infants.[7,8] The decline is not unlikely to be due to iron deficiency since for instance

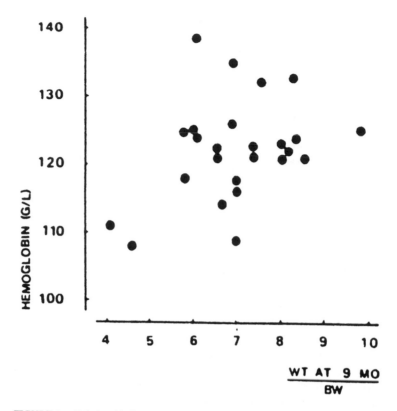

FIGURE 4.   Relationship between hemoglobin concentration and growth rate in very low birth weight infants.[4] Hemoglobin at age 9 months and weight development during the first 9 months were compared. There was no correlation indicating that infants who grow faster are able to increase their absorption of iron, respectively.

TABLE 2
Hemoglobin Concentration in 6 Very Low-Birth-Weight Infants Without and in 22 Infants With Blood Transfusions During the First 2 Months of Life[4]

Age in months	Without transfusions	With transfusions
Birth	18.8 ± 1.1 (6)	16.0 ± 0.7 (21)
1	11.5 ± 1.0 (5)	11.8 ± 0.4 (21)
2	9.1 ± 0.5 (6)	9.5 ± 0.4 (22)
3	9.3 ± 0.3 (4)	8.8 ± 0.4 (20)
4	10.9 ± 0.3 (6)	10.1 ± 0.3 (19)
9	12.2 ± 0.1 (6)	12.2 ± 0.2 (20)
15	13.1 ± 0.4 (6)	13.0 ± 0.2 (18)

Note: The mean values (g/dl) ± SE are shown together with the number of subjects in parentheses.

differences in MCV values were found when comparing low-birth-weight infants receiving iron supplementation with those receiving no such supplementation during the first 2 months of life.[2] It has been suggested that the decline in MCV after birth may be the result of an aging red blood cell population in the face of the shortened red blood cell survival and bone marrow erythroid hypoplasia that are common at this age.[9]

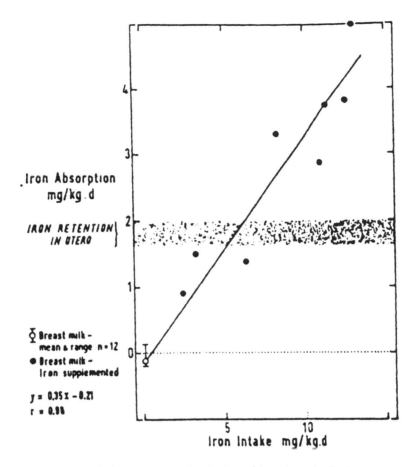

FIGURE 5. Relationship between iron intake and iron absorption in six preterm infants who received no blood transfusion.[6]

D. ROLE OF VITAMIN E AND SELENIUM

A documented metabolic role of vitamin E is the protection of biological membranes against oxidative breakdown of lipids. Premature infants' diet rich in polyunsaturated fatty acids, particularly when the diet is supplemented with iron, can produce a hemolytic anemia if vitamin E deficiency is not prevented or corrected (Figure 6). Melhorn and Gross[10] have demonstrated that in very low-birth-weight infants daily administration of 7 to 10 mg of iron per kilogram per day accelerated the postnatal decline in the concentration of hemoglobin. Williams et al.[11] observed increased hemolysis and lower hemoglobin levels in small prematures fed formulas with a high polyunsaturated fatty acid content especially when the formulas were fortified with iron.

Melhorn and Gross[12] have explored the relationship between gestational age and absorption of vitamin E. It is clear from their studies that during the first 3 weeks of life, infants with birth weight of less than 1500 g and gestational age of less than 32 weeks have low absorption of vitamin E. A subsequent study with a water soluble vitamin E preparation demonstrated a better absorption, but the individual levels were not predictable. Greaber et al. showed that vitamin E sufficiency, as defined by serum tocopherol levels and hydrogen peroxidase hemolysis tests, can be achieved rapidly and safely by the administration of intramuscular dl-α-tocopherol.[13] Analysis of their results indicate that a total intramuscular dose of vitamin E of 125 mg/kg administered over the first week of life is sufficient to meet vitamin E requirements during the first 6 weeks of life, even in the presence of intramuscular iron. Aside from mild erythema at the injection site, no detectable toxicity

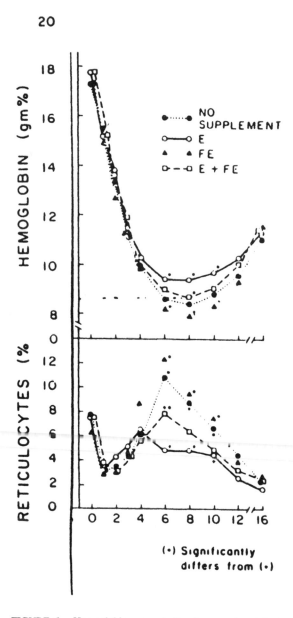

FIGURE 6.   Hemoglobin concentration in premature infants with a birth weight of 1000 to 1500 g. The infants were assigned to one of the four groups as follows: A, no additional supplement; B, ferrous sulfate, 8 mg of iron per kilogram per day up to 6 weeks of age; C, α-tocopherol acetate 25 IU/d between 2 and 6 weeks of age; D, both ferrous sulfate and α-tocopherol acetate.[10] The highest hemoglobin concentrations were in the vitamin E supplemented infants.

was related to vitamin E administration; however, Phelps[14] has in his recent article also emphasized potential dangers of vitamin E therapy.

Rudolph et al. have tested the role of selenium status in low-birth-weight infants fed formulas with and without iron. Under the conditions of their study, there was no evidence of any association between selenium values and early anemia of prematurity.[15]

E. INTERRELATIONSHIP WITH COPPER

Copper deficiency may occasionally occur in conditions where copper intake is minimal, for instance after prolonged parenteral nutrition if no copper is given. The question is whether copper deficiency exists in infants after preterm delivery and, if so, whether it has any influence on iron metabolism under these conditions. It has been demonstrated that the serum concentrations of copper are lower in preterm than full-term infants during the first months after birth.[16] It is difficult, however, to estimate the significance of this finding. It should be cautioned that any form of copper supplementation in formula-fed infants, if it ever proves to be indicated, leads to another problem since the amount of copper ingested is primarily dependent on the copper concentration of the water that is added to powdered formula. The concentration of copper in water is extremely variable in different areas and even between houses within a city particularly if the water supply comes from a private well. These problems are avoided if copper-supplemented ready-to-feed formulas are used.

Plasma levels of albumin and ceruloplasmin are low in very low-birth-weight infants compared to those found in term infants.[18,19] Both proteins are active in copper transport. Serum albumin is involved in the transport of ingested copper to the liver and ceruloplasmin in copper donation to extrahepatic tissues.[20] Hågå and Kran have shown that neither ceruloplasmin nor copper, zinc-superoxide dismutase activity seem to play a role in the etiology of the early anemia of prematurity.[19]

F. ROLE OF ERYTHROPOIETIN IN HEMATOPOIESIS

Maternal plasma concentration of erythropoietin tends to increase during pregnancy.[21] It is unlikely that the maternal erythropoietin would leak into the fetus through placental transfer.[22] Thus, the erythropoietin detected by some authors in cord blood samples even at early gestation is probably produced by the fetus itself.[23] Thomas et al. have detected a linear correlation between erythropoietin concentration and gestational age (Figure 7). Further, responses in erythropoietin levels were seen after severe anemia and intrauterine transfusion from 24 weeks gestation.[23]

Some data indicate that production of erythropoietin might be stimulated by secretion of insulin[24] and in conditions of placental insufficiency.[25]

G. DOES PROTEIN INTAKE LIMIT THE DEVELOPMENT OF HEMOGLOBIN CONCENTRATION IN HUMAN MILK-FED VERY LOW-BIRTH-WEIGHT INFANTS?

Human milk contains much less protein than cow milk or industrially produced infant milk formulas. Further, a 20 to 30% proportion of the milk nitrogen is nonprotein nitrogen.[26,27] Some evidence further indicates that a part of the actual protein in human milk is not bioavailable to infants. Such proteins may be lactoferrin and IgA in milk.[28] After these considerations, one may estimate that average human milk contains as low as 0.75 g of available protein per deciliter. Further, individual healthy women may secrete milk which contains only 0.5 g/dl of total protein. Thus, all exclusively human milk-fed infants or prematures receive relatively little protein, and in some cases the protein intake may be very small. It would not be surprising if the protein intake would be marginal particularly in very low-birth-weight infants.[26-30]

Results of a recent study indicate that protein intake is a rate-limiting factor which determines the concentration level of hemoglobin in human milk-fed very low-birth-weight infants during their 2nd and 3rd months of life.[31] A serious possibility is that the very low-birth-weight infants, fed human milk, suffer from real protein malnutrition. Consequently, impaired globin synthesis might be a rate-limiting factor in hemoglobin synthesis. General hypoproteinemia[29] and slow growth[30] found in human milk-fed very low-birth-weight infants would also fit with the possibility of nutritional protein deficiency. Further, it has been

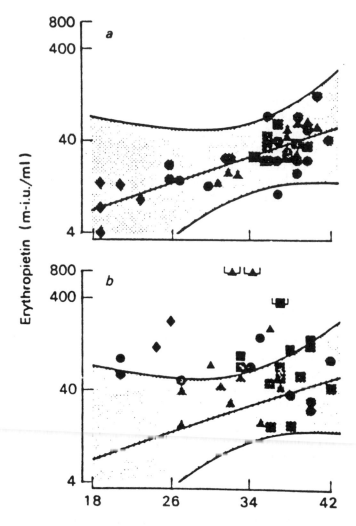

FIGURE 7.   Estimates of cord serum erythropoietin and gestation in normal (upper) and abnormal (lower) pregnancy. ●, vaginal delivery; ■, forceps; ▲, cesarean section; ◆, fetoscopy. The solid line shows the predicted value and the shaded area represents the 95% confidence band for single observations of erythropoietin in normal pregnancy.[23]

shown that after supplementing milk with protein isolated from human milk, the hemoglobin concentration increased significantly in very low-birth-weight infants.[31] Quantitatively, this increase elevated the mean hemoglobin concentration of the very low-birth-weight infants up to the normal range of full-term infants[4,31] (Figure 8). In fact, even the range of the values was practically similar to the full-term infants, as also demonstrated in Figure 9. This is the first demonstration that premature and full-term infants could have similar developmental changes in their hemoglobin concentration if the prematures are adequately fed and given enough protein of adequate quality.[31] If so, the concept would indirectly suggest that human milk protein in excess is better than a respective amount of nonhuman protein; however, there are no data directly supporting this possibility.

The influence of protein supplementation on hemoglobin concentration was not due to blood transfusions. In this study, the preterm infants treated with exchange transfusion after birth and those who received blood transfusions after age 6 weeks were excluded. In this way, infants in whom red cell transfusions were used to compensate for blood samples drawn for laboratory investigations were included, and those who developed anemia later,

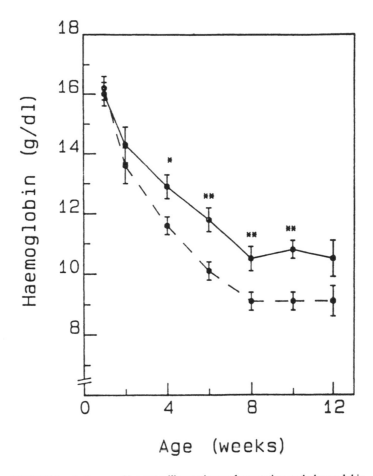

FIGURE 8. Influence of human milk protein supplementation on the hemoglobin concentration in very low-birth-weight infants.[31] The supplementation doubled the average daily protein intake of the infants: ———, supplemented; — — —, unsupplemented infants.

for other reasons, were excluded.[31] The observation was also essentially similar if we analyzed only the results from infants who had not undergone transfusion. The mean concentrations of hemoglobin were statistically different at 4 ($p < 0.05$) and 6 weeks of age ($p < 0.001$). Individual values are shown in Figure 10.[31]

It is interesting that the reticulocytosis started about 2 weeks earlier in the human milk protein-supplemented very low-birth-weight infants than in those fed with plain human milk.[31] The values also peaked and ceased earlier (Figure 11). Figure 12 shows the correlation between individual concentrations of hemoglobin at age 8 weeks and total serum protein at age 4 weeks in all infants. The correlation was also similar with regard to hematocrit values and red blood cell counts.[31] This observation further supports the possibility that the lack of protein represents a real phenomenon which can be corrected by adding human milk protein in the nutrition of very low-birth-weight infants even soon after birth.

Kumar et al.[17] have studied the effect of progressive protein deprivation in the monkey to determine which laboratory tests are affected early and which reflect the severity of protein deprivation. They found reduced hematocrit values after 4 weeks of protein deprivation. Total serum protein and transferrin were affected later, from 6 to 16 weeks and seemed to reflect the severity of protein deprivation. Rönnholm et al.[31] found low levels of total serum protein, transferrin, hematocrit, erythrocytes, and hemoglobin as early as age 4 weeks in protein-unsupplemented infants. This phenomenon is in accordance with the even greater need to use protein for growth in these very low-birth-weight infants.

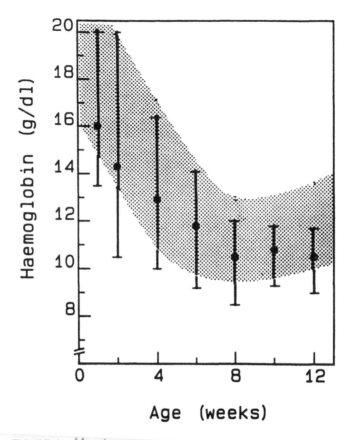

FIGURE 9.   Mean hemoglobin concentration (and total range) of very
low-birth-weight infants who were supplemented with human milk protein.[31] The shaded area represents the 95% range of hemoglobin concentration in healthy full-term infants.

Evidence of hemolysis has been shown in children with protein-energy malnutrition.
The hemolysis may be caused by low activity of superoxide dismutase and glutathione
peroxidase enzymes in erythrocytes. Decreased activities of these enzymes seem also to be
related to a reduced availability of copper and selenium. In a study of Rudolf et al., however,
an early decline in the concentration of hemoglobin did not correlate with red blood cell
selenium values or gluthathione peroxidase activity in very low-birth-weight infants.[15] In
another study design, the intake of selenium and the subsequent concentration of red blood
cell selenium were dependent on protein intake in low-birth-weight infants given either
human milk or human milk supplemented with human protein. Thus, it is not surprising
that both intakes correlated with hemoglobin concentrations even if the authors feel that the
weaker correlation with selenium is a secondary phenomenon. The patterns of reticulocyte
counts in these infants are also evidence against any hemolysis in the unsupplemented infants
as discussed later.

H. GROWTH AND IRON NEEDS

During the last 10 years, there has been a remarkable development in survival of very
low-birth-weight infants. Table 3 shows a schematic comparison of iron nutrition between
such a very low-birth-weight infant and large newborns. The calculations indicate that a
full-term infant who grows from 3.2 kg at birth to 10 kg at 1 year of age increases his total
body iron from 210 to 365 mg. Thus, the estimated increase in total body iron is about 50%
although the body weight triples during the same time. A very low-birth-weight infant with

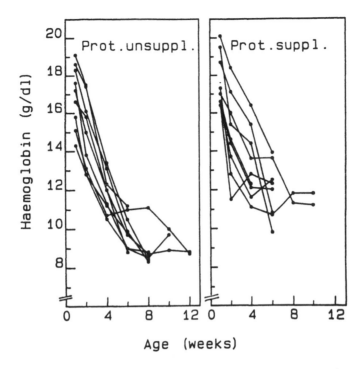

FIGURE 10. Hemoglobin concentrations in human milk protein supplemented very low-birth-weight infants. Only the untransfused infants are included[31]

a birth weight of 0.8 kg may increase his weight tenfold during the first year. If the respective rise in total body iron is calculated, the figures show that the infant has about 50 mg of iron at birth and 260 mg at 1 year of age, indicating a fivefold increase in total body iron. These numbers clearly show that the body weight increments are not in linear correlation with total body iron increments. The actual correlation indicates that the need for iron in very rapidly growing low-birth-weight infants is larger than one would estimate by the change in body weight. Table 3 indicates that the change in body iron per 12 months is similar in a case where the birth weight is 0.8 kg, 1.6 kg, or 3.2 kg. However, the smaller infants eat less than the larger infants and they must obtain their iron from a smaller volume of food, which may not be possible with a similar degree of iron supplementation.

III. HEMATOPOIESIS IN FULL-TERM INFANTS

A. MATERNAL-FETAL RELATIONSHIPS

Pregnancy is a period of increased need for dietary iron; however, the consequences of iron deficiency affect the mother far more than the fetus. In the fetus, the ratio of iron to body weight remains relatively constant throughout pregnancy at an average level of 75 mg/kg (Figure 13). The iron requirements of pregnancy during the latter half of pregnancy are high, and iron deficiency anemia is common in the mother, particularly during the end of pregnancy. With few exceptions, however, comparisons of iron-deficient and iron-sufficient mothers not only show that the hemoglobin concentrations of their offspring are indistinguishable at birth, but that they remain so during the remainder of the first year of life.

In one study, serum ferritin and blood hemoglobin concentrations were determined in 103 pregnant women and in cord blood of their normal full-term offspring. The relationships between maternal and infant iron status were investigated in detail. In 50 of the cases, placental non-heme iron was also measured.[32] The authors found an inverse relationship

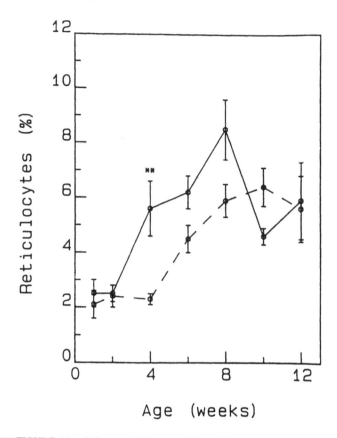

FIGURE 11.   Influence of human milk protein supplementation on reticulocyte count in human milk-fed very low-birth-weight infants:[51] ——, supplemented; — — —, unsupplemented infants.

between cord serum ferritin and hemoglobin concentrations (Figure 14) and speculated that the amount of iron in fetal stores is influenced by that required for hemoglobin synthesis. It is interesting that the maternal iron reserves, as estimated by their serum ferritin concentrations, were shown to be associated to the amount of non-heme iron in the placenta (Figure 15).

B. DEVELOPMENTAL CHANGES IN HEMOGLOBIN CONCENTRATION OF FULL-TERM INFANTS

It is difficult to determine hemoglobin concentration accurately soon after birth. Nevertheless, the level is highest during normal human development (Table 4). After birth, hemoglobin concentration decreases to values around 9 to 11 g/dl by the age of around 2 months. This period is followed by stimulated erythropoiesis which first stops the decline of hemoglobin concentration and then leads to a gradual and slow rise of hemoglobin to a mean value of about 11 g/dl with a range from 10 to 12 g/dl by about 6 months of age and to a mean of 11.5 g/dl (10.5 to 12.5 g/dl) by age about 12 months. This development is provided by adequate supply of nutritional iron. The use of iron-unsupplemented formulas with unsupplemented beikost may result in lower hemoglobin concentrations at and after age 4 months due to marginal iron deficiency which limits the optimal development of hemoglobin synthesis.[33] Under these conditions, a response in hemoglobin concentration may be achieved by a course of medicinal iron tablets, indicating that a small decrease of hemoglobin concentration may be an early sign of iron lack. It may also be true that some iron excess, even under physiological conditions, results in a reverse phenomenon. It has

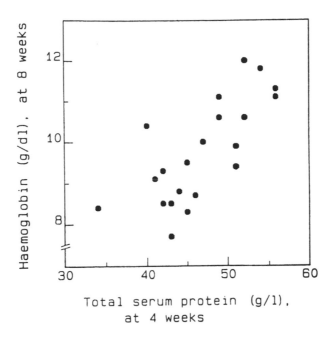

FIGURE 12.   Correlation between the hemoglobin concentration (at
age 8 weeks) and the preceding total serum protein concentration at
age 4 weeks (r = 0.74, p <0.001).[31]

TABLE 3
Influence of Growth on Estimated Iron Needs
in Infants with Weights from 0.8 to 3.2 kg

	Increments in 12 months		
Initial birth weight (kg)	Body weight (kg)	Body iron (mg)	Ratio iron/weight (mg/kg)
0.8	7.2	210	29
1.6	7.9	215	27
3.2	6.8	155	23

been reported, within the normal range of hemoglobin concentration, that the hemoglobin concentration is dependent on transferrin iron saturation of the plasma in iron sufficient infants (Table 5).[35] Perhaps the strongest evidence for the relationship is data for the 2-month-old infants (Figure 16). At this age, a high serum ferritin concentration reflects abundant iron stores. The 95% range for serum ferritin concentration was from 80 to 400 ng/ml.[36] Similarly, the 95% range for transferrin iron saturation was from 21 to 63%, above the range associated with iron deficiency anemia in infants. Thus, there is no reason to suspect a lack of iron either in individual infants or in 2-month-old infants as a group to explain the relationship between transferrin iron saturation and hemoglobin concentration.[35]

There is a well-documented racial difference between blacks and whites in their mean hemoglobin concentration. Although more detailed studies are lacking in infants, a large American survey (NHANES I) showed a difference also at age 1 year.[37] In 110 pairs of infants, the difference in hemoglobin concentration was 1.0 g/dl in populations which were income-matched and included all transferrin iron saturation levels. The difference was 0.7 g/dl if low transferrin iron saturations were excluded, and was not statistically significant.[37] The results from the same survey also suggested that the hemoglobin concentration is slightly

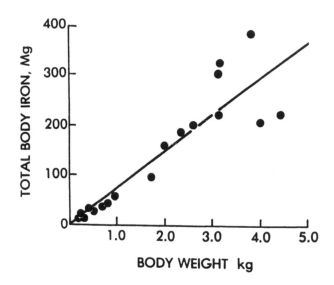

FIGURE 13.   Iron content and body weight in the fetus and newborn child.[49]

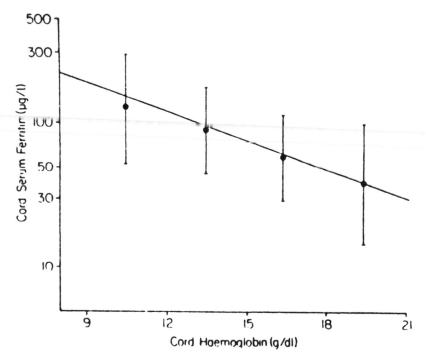

FIGURE 14.   The relationship between hemoglobin and serum ferritin concentrations in cord blood (r = −0.35, p <0.001).[32]

but consistently higher in obese infants than lean infants. The difference in mean values was 0.3 g/dl in boys and 0.12 g/dl in girls.[38] This trend remained unaltered if transferrin iron saturations below 16% were excluded from the data. The authors speculate that the finding may be explained by higher food intake for the obese than the lean, but there may also be additional explanations as in the polycythemia of the massively obese.[38]

C. EXCLUSIVE BREAST FEEDING AND HEMATOPOIESIS
Prolonged more or less exclusive breast feeding is practiced by many mothers in hope to improve health or to prevent diseases. Prolonged and exclusive breast feeding is a unique

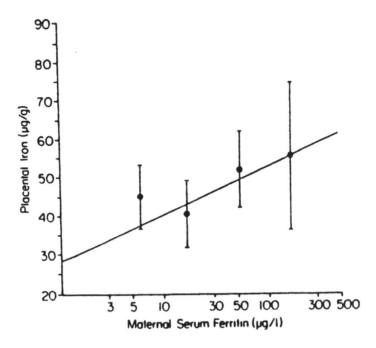

FIGURE 15. The relationship between maternal serum ferritin concentration and the concentration of non-heme iron in the placenta (r = 0.41, p <0.005).[32]

TABLE 4
Hemoglobin Concentrations in Iron-Supplemented Full-Term Infants[34]

Age (months)	(n)	Hemoglobin (g/dl) mean ± SEM	± 2 SD
0.5	(232)	16.6 ± 0.11	13.4—19.8
1	(240)	13.9 ± 0.10	10.7—16.1
2	(241)	11.2 ± 0.06	9.4—13.0
4	(52)	12.2 ± 0.14	10.3—14.1
6	(52)	12.6 ± 0.10	11.1—14.1
9	(56)	12.7 ± 0.09	11.4—14.0
15	(56)	12.7 ± 0.09	11.3—14.1

From Saarinen, V. M. and Siimes, M. A., *J. Pediatr.*, 92, 412, 1978. With permission.

model for human studies of erythropoiesis and iron requirement which has not been widely used. McMillan et al. were the first to report their findings on four infants in the U.S. who were exclusively breast fed for about 11 months. They found that all four infants had normal hemoglobin concentration, serum iron concentration, serum transferrin iron saturation, and erythrocyte protoporphyrin values, even though the infants had not, according to their history, received any supplemental or medicinal iron.[39] Pastel et al. obtained blood samples from seven healthy infants in the Peruvian Andes.[40] The infants had been exclusively breast-fed for 7.5 to 12 months. None had received supplemental water or iron prior to the examinations. The authors were unable to study hemoglobin concentration or red blood cell indices. They compared the serum ferritin and erythrocyte protoporphyrin values with those obtained from U.S. infants fed a variety of diets, with or without iron supplementation.

They found the values similar in the two groups. These studies suggest that exclusive

TABLE 5
Hemoglobin Concentration as a Function of Transferrin Saturation[35]

		Total group			After exclusion of transferrin saturation <16% or serum ferritin <10 ng/ml				
Age	(n)	Mean hemoglobin	Slope[a]	p	% Excluded	(n)	Mean hemoglobin	Slope[a]	p
2 mo	235	11.1	0.0134	<0.001	1	232	11.1	0.0124	k<0.005
4 mo	216	11.9	0.0128	<0.01	24	164	12.0	0.0110	NS[b]
6 mo	231	12.3	0.0212	<0.001	33	154	12.4	0.0146	<0.01
9 mo	230	12.4	0.0335	<0.001	30	161	12.6	0.0210	<0.01
12 mo	224	12.5	0.0241	<0.001	30	156	12.6	0.0188	<0.005

[a] Regression coefficient; hemoglobin, g/dl, per unit of transferrin saturation, %.
[b] Not significant.

From Siimes, M. A., Saarinen, V. M., and Dallman, P. R., *Am. J. Clin. Nutr.*, 32, 2295, 1979. With permission.

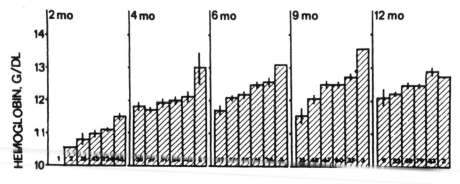

FIGURE 16.   Concentration of hemoglobin in various ranges of transferrin saturation from 2 through 12 months of age.[35] At each age, the ranges of the categories represented by bars from left to right were less than 10%, 10 to 16%, 16 to 22%, 22 to 30%, 30 to 50%, and above 50%. Mean values ± SEM of hemoglobin concentrations and number of subjects in each category are shown.

breast feeding is sufficient to maintain adequate iron nutrition for most, if not all, of the first year of life. This is an important conclusion with practical implications for large populations of infants, both in industrialized and nonindustrialized countries. However, this conclusion was based on direct and indirect evidence from a total of 11 infants who were not followed.

In a recent study, a group of 198 healthy, full-term infants were carefully followed.[41] All mothers were encouraged to breast-feed exclusively as long as possible. This resulted in 36 infants who were exclusively breast fed for 9 months without the use of any other food except some water and A-D vitamin drops. The 32 infants from the same series who were completely weaned prior to age 3.5 months served as their controls. The latter infants received iron supplementation through formula and solid foods. The results indicated that a great majority of exclusively breast fed infants were able to maintain their iron status at the same level as iron-supplemented controls. In fact, the mean concentration of hemoglobin was higher in the exclusively breast-fed infants than in controls at ages 4 and 6 months (Figure 17). This is an unexpected finding which is difficult to explain particularly since the phenomenon was independent of iron intake and iron nutrition of the infants. Further, the authors could not demonstrate any anemia in any individual infants, even after exclusive

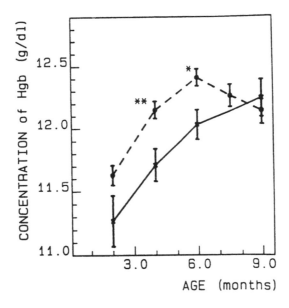

FIGURE 17. Concentration of hemoglobin in exclusively breast-fed infants without any iron supplementation (dashed line) and in control subjects who received iron-supplemented formula and solid foods after some breast feeding: x, $p < 0.005$, xx, $p < 0.01$.

breast feeding for 9 months. However, detailed analysis of the data showed a shift of the distribution of other laboratory criteria toward the lower limits of normal. This indicates that the risk of developing iron deficiency, although it is relatively small by 9 months in this population, increases as exclusive breast feeding is prolonged.[41] The results further indicated that maternal iron supplementaion during exclusive breast feeding even in large daily doses of 266 mg did not have any effect on the infants' iron nutrition, or prevent infants developing some laboratory signs of iron deficiency.[41] This observation is in accordance with another recent study in which the authors found no correlation between iron concentration in human milk and maternal iron stores.[42]

IV. MEASURES OF IRON STORES IN INFANTS

A. DOES SERUM FERRITIN ALSO MEASURE IRON STORES IN INFANTS?

There is documentation that the concentration of serum ferritin reflects the size of iron stores accurately in healthy adults and, with certain exceptions, also in adults with several disorders or diseases. The strongest evidence is based on studies where the individual concentration of serum ferritin was followed in healthy subjects after repeated phlebotomies.[43] The serum ferritin decreased as might be anticipated. There are also several studies in which serum ferritin concentrations have been compared with respective bone marrow iron or liver iron, or followed in patients who receive multiple blood transfusions. All this and similar other evidence indicate that serum ferritin concentration is, in fact, the best available single criterion of the size of iron stores or that of available iron stores.

Among infants, there is no direct evidence that serum ferritin concentrations function similarly as in adults although several indirect pieces of data suggest that it might; however, there are also observations which do not fit in this concept.

The first study on serum ferritin in infants was published in 1974.[44] It showed that in a California population of healthy infants, the concentration of serum ferritin was considerably higher in cord blood samples than in adult females (Figure 18). On the other hand,

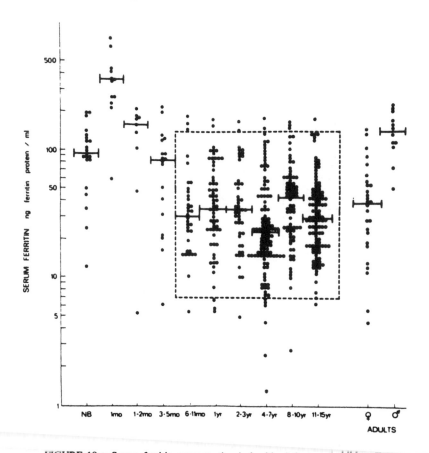

FIGURE 18.   Serum ferritin concentration in healthy infants and children.[44]

the newborn levels were similar to those of adult males.[44] There was a large individual variation of values at birth even if no low values were found. In fact, all concentrations were far above the mean level of for instance healthy females. The ferritin concentration was even higher at age 2 weeks than at the time of birth. The rise represented a more than doubling of the mean level and resulted in values above those found in healthy males and far above those in females. The study also showed that serum ferritin values gradually decreased during the next 6 months to low levels which were similar to or lower than those found in healthy females, and remained so through the infancy period (Figure 18).[44] Similar patterns of serum ferritin concentration have been observed in many subsequent studies.[45] This pattern of changes fits what might be expected to occur in the tissue iron stores of healthy infants. Supportive evidence is also obtained from groups of infants with iron deficiency anemia who do have low serum ferritin. The infants have elevated serum ferritin after blood transfusions.[44] However, during the natural development of mild iron deficiency, serum ferritin may remain within normal limits even if there is some other independent evidence of iron deficiency.[45] Also in low-birth-weight infants, anemia may appear prior to the depletion of serum ferritin.[2]

It is interesting that the early work of Smith et al.[46] showed that the total iron content of liver decreased relatively slowly in infants (Table 6). Their mean values were 1.3, 0.9, and 0.4 mg Fe/10 g of liver tissue at age groups of 0 to 6 months, 6 to 12 months, and 12 to 24 months, respectively. The values for water insoluble iron content had a similar pattern although the actual mean values were about half of the total iron (Table 6). Thus, the lowest level of liver iron was reached during the 2nd year of life. This is roughly about 12 months later than the age when serum ferritin concentration reaches its average minimum in any

TABLE 6
Liver Iron in Infants and Small Children: An Autopsy Material[46]

Age group (months)	(n)	Liver tissue (mg Fe per 10 g)		
		Mean value	Highest concentration	Lowest concentration
Total Iron Content				
0—6	14	1.3	1.6	0.6
6—12	10	0.9	1.2	0.6
12—24	7	0.4	0.7	0.3
24—40	16	0.6	1.0	0.3
Water Soluble Iron Content				
0—6	14	0.5	0.7	0.09
6—12	10	0.5	0.5	0.2
12—24	7	0.2	0.2	0.1
24—40	16	0.3	0.5	0.1

From Smith, N. J., Rosello, S., Say, M. B., and Yeya, K., *Pediatrics*, 16, 166, 1955. With permission.

group of healthy infants.[36,44,45] This piece of evidence also suggests that average serum ferritin concentration may not vary with liver iron.

These findings and others like them may be stated as evidence against serum ferritin as a measure of iron stores in infants since they do not fit the classical hypothesis of development of iron deficiency. A hypothetical reason could be that the iron stores of the fetus, representing about one third of the total body iron at the time of birth, would consist of isoferritins which are not specifically detectable by the routine serum ferritin assays. Other explanations may also be given as discussed later. Nevertheless, in the following discussion, we do consider serum ferritin concentration usable as a measure of iron stores also in infants.

It was soon obvious that ferritin values of 200 to 400 ng/ml cannot quantitatively represent a similar amount of storage iron in a healthy newborn infant and an adult male even if it is a common and average value in both. Some evidence was shown that there is an excellent correlation between serum ferritin and storage iron if the storage iron is expressed as concentration of iron[47] as shown also in Figure 19. A similar correlation has also been reported by calculation of iron stores at age 12 weeks (Figure 20)[48] Thus, storage iron cannot be estimated by 8 ng/ml to represent 1 mg[49] in young children.

B. FETAL SERUM FERRITIN

It is well documented that the fetus accumulates iron into its iron stores during pregnancy. It has been estimated that the amount of this iron is about 15 mg/kg by the time of birth. There seems to be a roughly linear correlation between the body weight and the quantity of total body iron.[50] The data from the fetuses and newborns showed a gradual increase in the concentrations of serum ferritin throughout the pregnancy.[51,52] The median value of early fetal samples at 14 to 16 weeks of gestation was 45 µg/l, with a range from 30 to 60 µ/l.[52] By the 39th week of gestation, the respective median value had gradually increased to about 200 µg/l, with a total range from 100 to 370 µg/l. The values of all these subjects, throughout pregnancy, are shown in Figure 21. The concentration of serum ferritin did not correlate with the placental weight or the birth weight.[52-54] The results, however, indicated a gradual

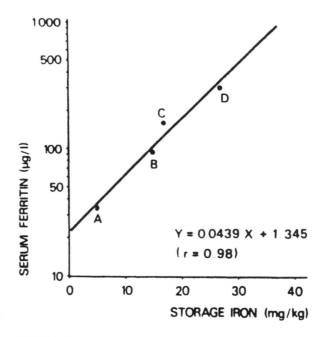

FIGURE 19.   Linear regression of four paired mean values of serum ferritin and iron stores per kilogram of body weight. A, adult females; B, adult males; C, newborn infants; D, calculated values from 2 week old infants.[47]

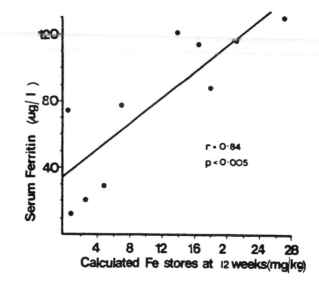

FIGURE 20.   Correlation between serum ferritin concentration and calculated iron stores at age 12 weeks (mg/kg).[48]

rise in the amount of fetal storage iron as the gestational age increases. Another study of 69 low-birth-weight infants indicated that serum ferritin values at age 24 to 48 h would be more representative of iron stores at birth than cord blood values.[51] The maternal ferritin concentration which may be influenced by parity and social class does not appear to control directly the fetal ferritin level.[53] Jansson et al. studied mothers of 20 normal infants[51] of which the concentration of serum ferritin was below 12 μg/l in four mothers. The infants of these mothers were divided into two groups: maternal ferritin <12 μg/l (A); maternal

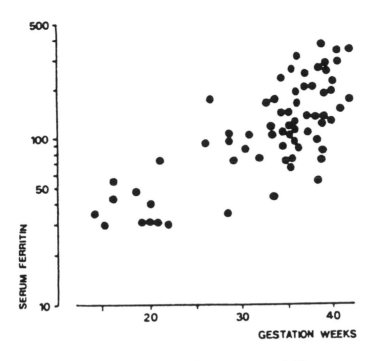

FIGURE 21. Serum ferritin (μg/l) in fetuses, preterm, and full-term new-borns.[52] The values are from cord blood samples.

ferritin >12 μg/l (B) (Figure 22). The serum ferritin level was similar in both groups and did not vary with that of the mothers.

A recent study on twins showed that there were only 4 out of 40 serum ferritin values which were not within the range of singletons indicating that iron stores are similar in singletons and twins.[52] This observation would also suggest that placental transfer of iron does not only compensate the need of iron for hemoglobin production, but also is capable of guaranteeing similar storage iron in twins as in singletons. This finding may also indicate that the subsequent risk of developing iron deficiency during the period of infancy would be similar in singletons and twins. This study further showed that the concentration of serum ferritin was similar (the difference between the two mean values being less than 30 μg/l) in half of the pairs of the twins.[52] This finding may indicate that there is a common tendency for similar amounts of storage iron to develop in both fetuses. The twin model allowed a good method to investigate the role of intrauterine growth retardation in the accumulation of storage iron since the gestational age was same in both infants.[52] It seems that intrauterine growth retardation slightly decreases, if anything, the concentrations of serum ferritin in the respective twin, partially decreasing the possibility that the twins have a similar concentration. On the other hand, in this study, the phenomenon was not consistent or impressive. However, there is another study indicating that serum ferritin may be lower in growth retarded new-borns.[51,55] In most studies, there was no correlation between the maternal concentration of serum ferritin and the newborn values. This finding indicates that maternal iron status has no important role in the regulation of iron accumulation into the fetal stores.[51,52,56-58] In contrast to these results, there are also some data indicating a weak correlation between maternal and fetal ferritin levels at delivery.[59,60] Thus, it is unlikely that the accumulation of fetal iron stores is regulated by the fetus itself, or by maternal iron metabolism. It has been speculated that the placenta or this circulation may have a specific role in this regu-lation.[52,61] Transferrin was found to be localized on the site facing the intervillous space, on the surface of the microvilli of the synctiotrophoblasts, whereas ferritin was shown to

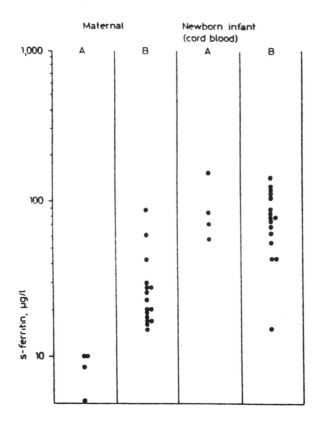

FIGURE 22.   Serum ferritin values in two groups of normal mothers at the time of delivery and the corresponding values for their newborn term infants. A, maternal serum ferritin <12 μg/l; B, maternal serum ferritin >12 μg/l.[51]

be present in all layers of the trophoblast and particularly in the synctiotrophoblast.[61] The authors postulate that human placental ferritin has the two functions of transporting iron when it is deficient and of storing it when it is present in excess. Ferritin appears to act as a safety valve in iron metabolism, regulating the transport of iron between mother and fetus and ensuring a constant supply of iron to the fetus.[61]

On the other hand, the independence of serum ferritin values in the newborn to those of the mother indicates that the fetus is capable of maintaining its own level of storage iron regardless of the maternal stores. Thus, the increase of maternal stores, for instance through iron medications prior to or during pregnancy, may not be reflected in the stores of the newborn. Further, one must emphasize that there are no data available indicating that a newborn with an unusually low serum ferritin value at or soon after birth, would be in an inferior position in regard to the likelihood of developing iron deficiency.

C. DEVELOPMENTAL CHANGES IN SERUM FERRITIN IN LOW-BIRTH-WEIGHT INFANTS

Prior to the use of serum ferritin assays, chemical data indicated a close correlation between iron content and body weight.[50] Similar conclusions were also made by investigating bone marrows of small prematures.[62]

Preterm infants have lower serum ferritin levels at and after birth than full-term infants.[51,55] Figure 23 shows changes in serum ferritin in a group of 28 infants between 29 and 37 weeks of gestational age compared to 19 full-term infants during 12 weeks after birth.[48]

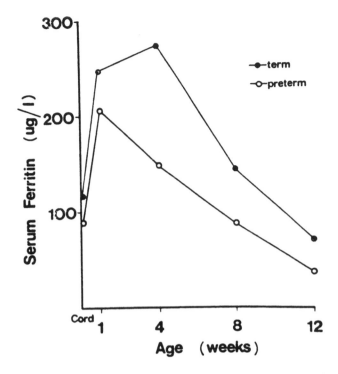

FIGURE 23. Mean serum ferritin concentration of infants at age 0 to 12 weeks: ○ = preterm infants, ● = term infants.[48]

D. MOBILIZATION OF STORAGE IRON

The high physiological concentration of hemoglobin at birth decreases to a lowest value at 2 months of age. This decrease in hemoglobin concentration initially results in a rise in tissue iron stores which are subsequently used during the next 12 months to maintain a normal level of hemoglobin. It seems that in each of the developmental changes of infancy there is a considerable individual variation, including the ability to mobilize iron from tissue stores. Thus, some infants may develop iron deficiency anemia even if they have iron stored in tissues (determined by their serum ferritin values) and having no disease, such as infection or inflammation, to explain the inability to mobilize iron stores.[45] A similar phenomenon may also occur in adults although only after significant blood loss. In contrast, in infants this phenomenon may be physiologic. In fact, in a large series of healthy infants who were followed carefully for their year of life, infants with mild iron deficiency anemia usually had serum ferritin concentration within normal range.[45] The relative abundance of storage iron in these cases may effectively inhibit the availability of iron from the other source, namely from intestinal absorption. Thus both sources of iron for hemoglobin synthesis, tissue stores and food, would be inhibited which coincidentally may subsequently increase the risk of developing iron deficiency anemia. Lundström et al. have also shown in preterm infants (Figure 24) that anemia commonly develops prior to the time when iron stores, as estimated by serum ferritin, are exhausted.[2] This latter finding also indicates that the rate at which iron can be mobilized from the tissues may not be fast enough in rapidly growing infants.

The mechanisms by which iron is mobilized from its tissue stores are not yet fully understood *in vivo*. Chelating agents are surprisingly ineffective in releasing iron from ferritin without reduction. Reducing agents, such as dithionite, thioglycolate, ascorbate, cysteine, and reduced glutathione may mobilize iron from ferritin *in vitro*.[63] Further, reduced flavins are effective in reducing ferritin iron under anaerobic conditions.[64] There is, however, no clear knowledge on the mechanisms in infants. The indirect evidence either based on serum

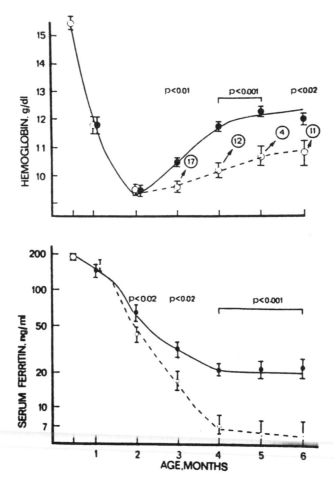

FIGURE 24. Hemoglobin concentration and serum ferritin concentration in low-birth-weight infants receiving no iron supplementation (○) or iron supplement of 2 mg/kg/d (●) starting at age 2 weeks.[2]

ferritin[2,36] or liver iron concentrations[46] suggests that iron from stores is released at a much slower rate in infants than in adults. Whether the iron stores carried by the fetus play a specific role remains to be determined.

E. SERUM FERRITIN IN FULL-TERM INFANTS

The physiological individuality of the serum ferritin values within the normal range suggests similar physiological "channels" for serum ferritin[36] as found for hemoglobin concentration and red blood cell indices.[45] Serum ferritin has proved to be a useful test in evaluating iron nutrition in groups of infants. The level of serum ferritin correlates well with iron intake, and low ferritin levels are associated with low transferrin saturation.[36] An unexpected finding has been a rise of the serum ferritin values during the latter half of infancy in many of the infants not supplemented with iron and with low serum ferritin values at 6 months of age.[36] One might speculate that the initially lower iron stores at 6 months of age and the subsequent follow-up without supplementation could induce enhanced absorption of iron and through this compensation even improve the iron status in many infants. However, this explanation is hypothetical and based on other studies indicating that depleted iron stores can enhance the bioavailability of iron.[65,66]

Serum ferritin is very low in infants with severe iron deficiency anemia.[45] Saarinen and

Siimes tried to evaluate the association between the low values of serum ferritin and other independent criteria of iron nutrition, such as hemoglobin concentration, MCV, and transferrin iron saturation in healthy infants.[36] One might expect to find either more abnormally low values or lower mean values of these parameters associated with low serum ferritin values in any population, if a ferritin value at the lower range of normal would reflect an amount of storage iron at the lower range. In fact, there was no difference either in hemoglobin, MCV, or transferrin iron saturation at 6 or 12 months of age in iron-supplemented infants with different levels of serum ferritin. However, in the iron-nonsupplemented healthy infants, there was a correlation between serum ferritin and transferrin iron saturation especially at 6 months of age. The infants with serum ferritin below -3 S.D. had a significantly lower transferrin iron saturation than the infants with serum ferritin above $+1$ S.D. There was no such correlation regarding the mean values of hemoglobin concentration or MCV.[36] These findings indicate that the serum ferritin concentration is surprisingly independent on other iron-related laboratory tests in healthy infants without any major iron deficiency. This same phenomenon has also demonstrated recently among 36 infants who received only human milk without any iron supplementation for the period of the first 9 months after birth.[41] Their average concentration of serum ferritin was 15 (13 to 17, $\pm$ SEM) μg/l compared to 27 (24 to 29, $\pm$ SEM) μg/l in infants receiving daily iron supplement at age 9 months. The upper range of the values were similar in both groups even if the mean values diverged.[41] This observation clearly shows that there are healthy individual infants who are able to maintain a similar concentration of serum ferritin regardless if they receive very little iron for 9 months or if they are supplemented daily for the same period of time.

F. ERYTHROCYTE FERRITIN

Porter[67] discovered that normal human red blood cells contain ferritin protein. More recently it has been documented that this ferritin is more reactive with antibody to heart ferritin than to spleen ferritin.[68] Further, adult data indicate that the erythrocyte ferritin might more sensitively measure some forms of storage iron since increased erythrocyte ferritin has been found in subjects with the β-thalassemia trait, though only in one case was the serum ferritin concentration higher than normal.[69] Peters et al. have followed an interesting adult patient with idiopathic hemochromatosis after weekly venesections (Figure 25). In this case, serum ferritin seems to decrease prior to the decrease in erythrocyte heart ferritin which may suggest that these ferritins reflect changes in different iron pools.[69] Unfortunately, little is known about erythrocyte ferritin patterns after birth and during infancy.

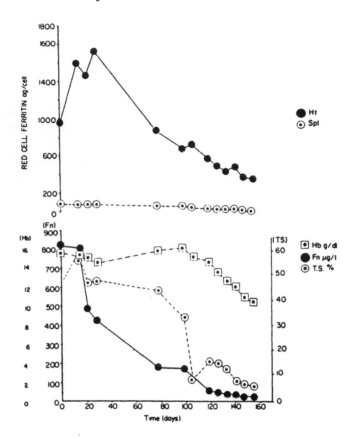

FIGURE 25.   Sequential changes in hematological status and serum ferritin (below) and erythrocyte heart (Ht) and spleen (Spl) ferritin concentrations (above) following the onset (day 0) of weekly venesection therapy in a case of idiopathic hemochromatosis.[69]

REFERENCES

1. **Wintrobe, M. M.,** *Clinical Hematology,* Lea & Febiger, Philadelphia, 1961.
2. **Lundström, U., Siimes, M. A., and Dallman, P. R.,** At what age does iron supplementation become necessary in low-birth-weight infants?, *J. Pediatr.,* 91, 878, 1977.
3. **Victorin, L. H. and Olegard, R.,** Iron in the preterm infant: a pilot study comparing Fe 2+ and Fe 3+ tolerance and effect, *J. Pediatr.,* 105, 151, 1984.
4. **Siimes, M. A. and Järvenpää, A-L.,** Prevention of anemia and iron deficiency in very low birth weight (VLBW) infants, *J. Pediatr.,* 101, 277, 1982.
5. **Lundström, U. and Siimes, M. A.,** Red blood cell values in low birth weight infants: ages at which values become equivalent to those of term infants, *J. Pediatr.,* 96, 1040, 1980.
6. **Shaw, J. C. L.,** Iron absorption by the premature infant, *Acta Paediatr. Scand. Suppl.,* 299, 83, 1982.
7. **Matoth, Y., Zaizov, R., and Varsano, I.,** Postnatal changes in some red cell parameters, *Acta Paediatr. Scand.,* 60, 317, 1971.
8. **Stockman, J. A.,** Anemia of prematurity, *Semin. Hematol.,* 12, 163, 1975.
9. **Stockman, J. A. and Oski, F. A.,** RBC values in low-birth-weight infants during the first seven weeks of life, *Am. J. Dis. Child.,* 134, 945, 1980.
10. **Melhorn, D. K. and Gross, S.,** Vitamin-E dependent anemia in the premature infant. I. Effects of large doses of medicinal iron, *J. Pediatr.,* 79, 569, 1971.

11. **Williams, M. L., Shott, R. J., O'Neal, P. L., and Oski, F. A.,** Role of dietary iron and fat on vitamin E deficiency anemia of infancy, *N. Engl. J. Med.,* 292, 887, 1975.

12. **Melhorn, D. K. and Gross, S.,** Vitamin-E dependent anemia in the premature infant. II. Relationships between gestational age and absorption of vitamin E, *J. Pediatr.,* 79, 581, 1971.

13. **Graeber, J. E., Williams, M. L., and Oski, F. A.,** The use of intramuscular vitamin E in the premature infant. Optimum dose and iron interaction, *J. Pediatr.,* 90, 282, 1977.

14. **Phelps, D. L.,** Vitamin E and retrolental fibroplasia in 1982, *Pediatrics,* 70, 420, 1982.

15. **Rudolph, N., Preis, O., Bitzos, E. I., Reale, M. M., and Wong, S. I.,** Hematologic and selenium status of low-birth-weight infants fed formula with and without iron, *J. Pediatr.,* 99, 57, 1981.

16. **Sann, L., Rigal, D., Galy, G., Bienvenu, F., and Bourgeois, J.,** Serum copper and zinc concentration in premature and small-for-date infants, *Pediatr. Res.,* 14, 1040, 1980.

17. **Kumar, V., Chase, H. P., Hammond, K., and O'Brien, D.,** Alterations in blood biochemical tests in progressive protein malnutrition, *Pediatrics,* 49, 736, 1972.

18. **Räihä, N. C. R., Heinonen, K., Rassin, D. K., and Gault, G. E.,** Milk protein quantity and quality in low-birth-weight infants. I. Metabolic responses and effect on growth, *Pediatrics,* 57, 659, 1976.

19. **Hågå, P. and Kran, S.,** Ceruloplasmin levels and erythrocyte superoxide dismutase activity in small preterm infants during the early anemia of prematurity, *Acta Paediatr. Scand.,* 70, 861, 1981.

20. **Evans, G. W.,** Copper homeostasis in the mammalian system, *Physiol. Rev.,* 53, 535, 1973.

21. **Cotes, P. M.,** Immunoreactive erythropoietin in serum. I. Evidence for the validity of the assay method and the physiological relevance of estimates, *Br. J. Haematol.,* 50, 427, 1982.

22. **Wasserman, R. R.,** Erythropoietin production in the fetus: role of the kidney and maternal anaemia, *J. Lab. Clin. Med.,* 83, 281, 1974.

23. **Thomas, R. M., Canning, C. E., Cotes, P. M., Linch, D. C., Rodeck, C. H., Rossiter, C. E., and Huehns, E. R.,** Erythropoietin and cord blood hemoglobin in the regulation of human fetal erythropoiesis, *Br. J. Obstet. Gynecol.,* 90, 795, 1983.

24. **Widness, J. A., Susa, J. B., Garcia, J. F., Singer, D. B., Segal, P., Oh, W., Schwartz, R., and Schwartz, H. C.,** Increased erythropoiesis and elevated erythropoietin in infants born to diabetic mothers and in hyperinsulinemic rhesus fetuses, *J. Clin. Invest.,* 67, 637, 1981.

25. **Meberg, A.,** Haemoglobin concentrations and erythropoietin levels in appropriate and small for gestational age infants, *Scand. J. Haematol.,* 24, 162, 1980.

26. **Hambraeus, L., Lönnerdal, B., Forsum, E., and Gebre-Medhin, M.,** Nitrogen and protein components of human milk, *Acta Paediatr. Scand.,* 67, 561, 1978.

27. **Lönnerdal, B. and Forsum, E.,** Casein content of human milk, *Am. J. Clin. Nutr.,* 41, 113, 1985.

28. **Jatzyk, G. V., Kuvaeva, I. B., and Gribakin, S. G.,** Immunological protection of the neonatal gastrointestinal tract: the importance of breast feeding, *Acta Paediatr. Scand.,* 74, 246, 1985.

29. **Rönnholm, K. A. R., Sipilä, I., and Siimes, M. A.,** Human milk protein supplementation for the prevention of hypoproteinemia without metabolic imbalance in breast milk-fed, very low-birth-weight infants, *J. Pediatr.,* 101, 243, 1982.

30. **Rönnholm, K. A. R.,** Human milk feeding in very low-birth-weight infants. Study on protein need, as estimated by growth, serum protein, aminoacid and hemoglobin concentrations and riboflavin status during the first year of life, Painovalssi, Helsinki, 1986, 1.

31. **Rönnholm, K. A. R. and Siimes, M. A.,** Haemoglobin concentration depends on protein intake in small preterm infants fed human milk, *Arch. Dis. Child.,* 60, 99, 1985.

32. **MacPhail, A. P., Charlton, R. W., Bothwell, T. H., and Torrance, J. D.,** The relationship between maternal and infant iron status, *Scand. J. Haematol.,* 25, 141, 1980.

33. **Saarinen, U. M.,** Need for iron supplementation in infants on prolonged breast feeding, *J. Pediatr.,* 93, 177, 1978.

34. **Saarinen, U. M. and Siimes, M. A.,** Developmental changes in red blood cell counts and indices of infants after exclusion of iron deficiency by laboratory criteria and continuous iron supplementation, *J. Pediatr.,* 92, 412, 1978.

35. **Siimes, M. A., Saarinen, U. M., and Dallman, P. R.,** Relationship between hemoglobin concentrations and transferrin saturation in iron-sufficient infants, *Am. J. Clin. Nutr.,* 32, 2295, 1979.

36. **Saarinen, U. M. and Siimes, M. A.,** Serum ferritin in assessment of iron nutrition in healthy infants, *Acta Paediatr. Scand.,* 67, 745, 1978.

37. **Garn, S. M., Ryan, A. S., Owen, D. G. M., and Abraham, S.,** Income matched black-white hemoglobin differences after correction for low transferrin saturations, *Am. J. Clin. Nutr.,* 34, 1645, 1981.

38. **Garn, S. M. and Ryan, A. S.,** The effect of fatness on hemoglobin levels, *Am. J. Clin. Nutr.,* 36, 189, 1982.

39. **McMillan, J. A., Landaw, S. A., and Oski, F. A.,** Iron sufficiency in breast-fed infants and the availability of iron from human milk, *Pediatrics,* 58, 686, 1976.

40. **Pastel, R. A., Howanitz, P. J., and Oski, F. A.,** Iron sufficiency with prolonged exclusive breast-feeding in Peruvian infants, *Clin. Pediatr.,* 20, 625, 1981.

41. **Siimes, M. A., Salmenperä, L., and Perheentupa, J.,** Exclusive breast-feeding for 9 months: risk of iron deficiency, *J. Pediatr.,* 104, 196, 1984.
42. **Celeda, A., Bussett, R., Gutierrez, J., and Herreros, V.,** No correlation between iron concentration in breast milk and maternal iron stores, *Helv. Paediatr. Acta,* 37, 11, 1982.
43. **Dauncey, M. J., Davies, C. G., Shaw, J. C. L., and Urman, J.,** The effect of iron supplements and blood transfusion on iron absorption by low birthweight infants fed pasteurized human breast milk, *Pediatr. Res.,* 12, 899, 1978.
44. **Siimes, M. A., Addiego, J. E., and Dallman, P. R.,** Ferritin in serum: diagnosis of iron deficiency and iron overload in infants and children, *Blood,* 43, 581, 1974.
45. **Dallman, P. R., Siimes, M. A., and Stekel, A.,** Iron deficiency in infancy and childhood, *Am. J. Clin. Nutr.,* 33, 86, 1980.
46. **Smith, N. J., Rosello, S., Say, M. B., and Yeya, K.,** Iron storage in the first five years of life, *Pediatrics,* 16, 166, 1955.
47. **Saarinen, U. M. and Siimes, M. A.,** Iron absorption from breast milk, cow's milk and iron-supplemented formula: an opportunistic use of changes in total body iron determined by hemoglobin, ferritin and body weight in 132 infants, *Pediatr. Res.,* 13, 143, 1979.
48. **Messer, R. D., Russo, A. M., McWhirter, W. R., Sprangemeyer, D., and Halliday, J. W.,** Serum ferritin in term and preterm infants, *Aust. Paediatr. J.,* 16, 185, 1980.
49. **Walters, G. O., Miller, F., and Worwood, M.,** Serum ferritin concentration and iron stores in normal subjects, *J. Clin. Pathol.,* 26, 770, 1973.
50. **Widdowson, E. M. and Spray, C. M.,** Chemical development *in utero, Arch. Dis. Child.,* 26, 205, 1951.
51. **Jansson, L., Holmberg, L., and Ekman, R.,** Variation of serum ferritin in low birth weight infants with maternal ferritin, birth weight and gestational age, *Acta Haematol.,* 62, 273, 1979.
52. **Siimes, A. S. I. and Siimes, M. A.,** Changes in the concentration of ferritin in the serum during fetal life in singletons and twins, *Early Hum. Dev.,* 13, 47, 1986.
53. **Kelly, A. M., MacDonald, D. J., and McDougall, A. N.,** Observations on maternal and fetal ferritin concentration at term, *Br. J. Obstet. Gynaecol.,* 85, 338, 1978.
54. **Bratlid, D. and Moe, P. J.,** Hemoglobin and serum ferritin levels in mothers and infants at birth, *Eur. J. Pediatr.,* 134, 125, 1980.
55. **Hågå, P.,** Plasma ferritin concentrations in preterm infants in cord blood and during the early anaemia of prematurity, *Acta Paediatr. Scand.,* 69, 637, 1980.
56. **Jansson, L., Holmberg, L., and Ekman, R.,** Variation of serum ferritin in low birth weight infants with maternal ferritin, birth weight and gestational age, *Acta Haematol.,* 62, 273, 1979.
57. **Rios, E., Lipschitz, D. A., Cook, J. D., and Smith, N. J.,** Relationship of maternal and infant iron stores as assessed by determination of plasma ferritin, *Pediatrics,* 55, 694, 1975.
58. **Wallenburg, H. C. S. and van Eijk, H. G.,** Effect of oral iron supplementation during pregnancy on maternal and fetal iron status, *J. Perinat. Med.,* 12, 7, 1984.
59. **Kaneshige, E.,** Serum ferritin as an assessment of iron stores and other hematologic parameters during pregnancy, *Obstet. Gynecol.,* 57, 238, 1981.
60. **Celada, A., Busset, R., Gutierrez, J., and Herreros, V.,** Maternal and cord blood ferritin, *Helv. Paediatr. Acta,* 37, 239, 1982.
61. **Okuyama, T., Tawada, T., Furuya, H., and Villee, C. A.,** The role of transferrin and ferritin in the fetal-maternal-placental unit, *Am. J. Obstet. Gynecol.,* 152, 344, 1985.
62. **Seip, M. and Halvorsen, S.,** Erythrocyte production and iron stores in premature infants during the first months of life, *Acta Paediatr. Scand.,* 45, 600, 1956.
63. **Pape, L., Multani, J. S., Stitt, C., and Saltman, P.,** The mobilization of iron from ferritin by chelating agents, *Biochemistry,* 7, 613, 1968.
64. **Sirivech, S., Frieden, E., and Osaki, S.,** The release of iron from horse spleen ferritin by reduced flavins, *Biochem. J.,* 143, 311, 1974.
65. **Heinrich, H. C., Gabbe, E. E., and Whang, D. H.,** Die Dosabhängigkeit der intestinalen Eisenresorption bei Menschen mit normalen Eisenreserven und Personen mit prälatentem/latentem Eisenmangel, *Z. Naturforsch.,* 24b, 1301, 1969.
66. **Walters, G. O.,** Iron stores and iron absorption, *Lancet,* 2, 1216, 1973.
67. **Porter, F. S.,** Erythrocyte ferritin, *Pediatr. Res.,* 7, 954, 1973.
68. **Jacobs, A., Peters, S. W., Bauminger, E. R., Eikelboom, J., Ofer, S., and Rachmilewitz, E. A.,** Ferritin concentration in normal and abnormal erythrocytes measured by immunoradiometric assay with antibodies to heart and spleen ferritin and Mössbauer spectroscopy, *Br. J. Haematol.,* 49, 201, 1981.
69. **Peters, S. W., Jacobs, A., and Fitzsimons, E.,** Erythrocyte ferritin in normal subjects and patients with abnormal iron metabolism, *Br. J. Haematol.,* 53, 211, 1983.

Chapter 3

NONHEMATOLOGICAL MANIFESTATIONS OF IRON DEFICIENCY

Helmut A. Huebers

TABLE OF CONTENTS

I. INTRODUCTION

Iron deficiency is present when body iron content is diminished.[1,2] The presence of iron deficiency implies neither the degree of depletion nor the presence of anemia. Iron deficiency anemia refers to a hematologic state resulting from iron deficiency. Its occurrence implies that body iron stores as present in ferritin and hemosiderin have been exhausted and the organism is in the last stages of serious iron depletion. Thus, an individual may be iron deficient without manifesting iron deficiency anemia. The converse, however, does not occur.[3]

Certainly the most important function of iron in the body is its role in oxygen transport and storage. Therefore, the consequences of iron deficiency have traditionally focused on anemia which reduces maximum oxygen consumption and maximum work performance.[4-6] Other consequences of iron deficiency anemia, especially in the severe forms, have been reported. These include shortened survival of erythrocytes in infants,[7] effects of anemia on serum total cholesterol and triglyceride levels,[8,9] reduced leukocyte alkaline phosphatase activity, decreased nitro-blue-tetrazolium (NBT) reduction ability, impaired liver growth, and generalized depression of DNA synthesis.[10] The latter may lead to increased fetal resorption, decreased fetal size, and a large decrease in total fetal weight in rats.[11-13] It has also been noted that rats with iron deficiency anemia show a significantly greater incidence of tongue tumors after exposure to carcinogen.[14]

Nonhematological manifestations related to iron deficiency have long been suspected but have generally been regarded as late and unusual complications of severe iron deficiency;[15-18] however, studies of Dallman and Siimes have shown that when iron supply to the erythron becomes inadequate, there is a depletion of essential iron in many other body tissues as well[19-21] (Figure 1). Because of the proportionality between the decrease in hemoglobin concentration and tissue iron, it is difficult to separate the effects of anemia per se and the more complex functional nonhematological consequences of iron deficiency. Recently, however, considerable progress has been made toward this distinction.[20,22] As will be learned, the major liabilities of tissue iron deficiency will lead to abnormalities in gastrointestinal function, work performance, neurological function, and immunity.[3,12,23-29] Aspects relating to immunity and/or infection are discussed in another chapter of this book. The purpose of this brief discussion is to summarize the effects of tissue iron deficiency and to call attention to the fact that iron deficiency is a systemic disease.

II. DETECTION OF IRON DEFICIENCY

Historically, attention in iron deficiency has been primarily directed to anemia for several reasons. (1) Most body iron, over 80% in iron-deficient individuals, is contained in the erythron; (2) a simple hemoglobin determination usually allows the recognition of the end stage of iron deficiency; and (3) the determination of iron concentration in other tissues would necessitate invasive sampling procedures. Accordingly, the hemoglobin concentration is extensively used as a yardstick for iron deficiency.[30] Because of the limited accuracy in the determination of blood volume, estimates of total iron based on hemoglobin concentration are highly subject to error.[31] Furthermore, because of the wide range of hemoglobin concentration found in nonanemic individuals, it may be possible to recognize that the value found in a given subject is indeed lower than it should be only after substantial iron deficiency has developed[32] (Figure 2). To adjust for these difficulties, especially in infants, it has been suggested to plot hemoglobin and red cell volume on percentile charts just as for height and weight.[30,32,33]

Recently, attention has shifted to more sensitive measurements of iron deficiency, including transferrin saturation with iron as an index of iron availability to tissues,[34,35] the

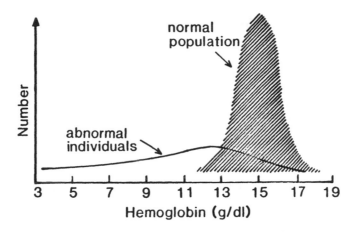

FIGURE 1. Distribution of normal and abnormal hemoglobin values. The hemoglobin values observed in a large population of normal individuals follows a symmetric (Gaussian) distribution. There is a considerable overlap between the normal population and abnormal individuals. The lower the hemoglobin value, the more likely it represents true anemia. Abnormal patients may not be detected because their hemoglobin value falls within the normal range.[32]

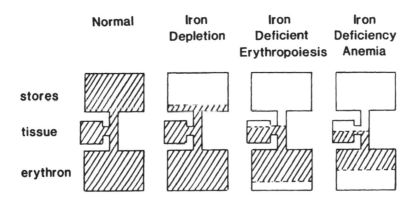

FIGURE 2. Schematic representation of the sequence of changes induced by a gradual reduction in the iron content of the body. Iron-containing tissue enzymes constitute a small but important compartment of iron amounting to 4 to 8 mg, and these enzymes are sensitive to changes in total body iron content.

serum ferritin concentration as a reflection of tissue iron stores,[36] and red cell protoporphyrin concentration which is increased when insufficient iron is being delivered to the red cell precursors to enable them to synthesize a full amount of hemoglobin.[2,16,37,38] By measurement of those laboratory parameters, it has been demonstrated that approximately 20% of the world's population is iron deficient and a much larger percentage is iron depleted.[16,39] Children are especially vulnerable to iron deficiency due to rapid growth, deficient dietary intake of iron, and blood loss.[40,41] In the U.S., the prevalence of iron deficiency anemia probably ranges between 5 and 20% among various age groups in childhood and adolescence.[19,42-44] The peak prevalence is between 6 months and 2 years of age. The high incidence of iron deficiency during adolescence, another period of rapid growth, has been appreciated only recently.[33,45] Half of the individuals who are iron deficient by chemical criteria have no demonstrable anemia.[44]

III. CLASSICAL SIGNS OF IRON DEFICIENCY

In the past, recognized tissue effects were largely anatomical. Koilonychia, or spoon-shaped nails, is listed in many medicine textbooks as almost diagnostic of iron deficiency. "Spooning" of the nails has been described in all age groups and this phenomenon has been seen in infants and children who are iron deficient and nonanemic. Trophic changes in iron deficiency may cause the hair to become brittle, splitting at the ends, and thinning, and there may also be early graying.[46] Atrophic rhinitis has been attributed to iron deficiency and can be relieved or cured by treatment with iron.[47,48] Another manifestation of iron deficiency appears to be generalized pruritis.[49]

Angular stomatitis, i.e., cracking and fissuring of the angles of the mouth, and glossitis, a condition in which the tongue is painful and red, have been noted in adults with iron deficiency and these epithelial changes show rapid clinical improvement following iron therapy.[46] These signs, however, are less specific for iron deficiency than koilonychia having been observed in a variety of other nutritional disturbances.

Dysphagia in iron deficiency anemia is believed to be secondary to obstruction caused by a web of tissues with a predilection for the postcricoid region of the hypopharynx. Webs can also occur in the esophagus; the specificity of web formation for iron deficiency has been questioned, however.[50,51] Moreover, in an iron-deficient individual, the esophageal web, which is a precancerous lesion, does not respond to iron therapy although dysphagia was frequently relieved.[52] It is also important to note that dysphagia is reported to be rare in parts of Africa in which iron deficiency is common.[53]

Dysphagia associated with atrophic changes in the tongue, fissures in the corner of the mouth, and predisposition to carcinoma in the region of the hypopharynx in the presence of iron deficiency is known as the Plummer-Vinson syndrome, or sideropenic dysphagia.[49] Although this syndrome was encountered many times, especially in women in the 1920s, it has virtually disappeared 4 decades later.[51] It has been suggested that a peculiarity of the diet (deficiency in fresh vegetables, fruits, and meat), consumed by the most affected group of women of Scandinavian descent in addition to iron deficiency, may have been a factor.[51]

Pica, a perversion of appetite characterized by the compulsive ingestion of nonfood substances, has been associated with iron deficiency anemia.[51,53] Pica is a frequent manifestation of iron deficiency in adults as well as children, occurring in more than 50% of children with iron deficiency in some series.[51] Iron-deficient individuals may crave any of a variety of substances, but many have an intense desire for ice ("pagophagia").[54] The craving for ice appears to be specific for iron deficiency and can be fully expressed in the absence of anemia. It could not be attributed to stomatitis or glossitis and was not satisfied by cold liquids or ice cream. Similarly, rats rendered iron deficient by bleeding were reported to exhibit a preference for ice rather than for water.[54] That pagophagia may be relieved by administration of iron has been observed long before modern times. Surprisingly, pagophagia is cured within a few days by the administration of very small amounts of iron, much less than those required to correct anemia or repair the iron store deficit.[51,55] Various other forms of pica have been observed in several parts of the world and occurs in at all ages but mostly in children and pregnant women. Subjects whose pica is characterized by the eating of clay or starch may have induced their own anemia, as these substances absorb iron and inhibit its absorption.[53]

Analysis of a large group of infants suggests that the iron-deficient infant is more commonly underweight for both age and height.[40,49] In 88 children, all of whom were less than 10 years of age, it was possible to ascertain weights at the time of recovery from the anemia. Infants whose rates of weight gain were decelerated prior to diagnosis, exhibited a rapid resumption of weight gain when iron therapy was instituted.[56] In addition, for infants who appeared to be growing normally, iron therapy may accelerate their rates of weight gain with iron supplements.

IV. GASTROINTESTINAL ABNORMALITIES

A relationship between iron deficiency and gastrointestinal abnormalities was noted as early as 1913, when it was noted that the atrophic gastritis observed in iron-deficient subjects was associated with a diminished secretion of gastric acid.[57] In addition to achlorhydria, which is the only well established impairment of the stomach in iron deficiency, other GI abnormalities are now recognized in infants and children with iron deficiency anemia.[53] These changes include xylose malabsorption, fat malabsorption, occult GI bleeding, an exudative enteropathy, beeturia, histological changes in the duodenal mucosa, and impairment of iron absorption.[49,51] Because reduced acid secretion by the stomach causes a pronounced impairment in the assimilation of dietary iron, it is not entirely clear whether chronic gastritis is the result or the cause of chronic iron deficiency. Most of the GI abnormalities listed above showed improvement after the institution of an iron therapy.[55] The malabsorption syndrome has been attributed to iron deficiency in growing children and this might explain the retarded growth that has been observed in the severely iron-deficient child.[49] However, the complexity of the clinical setting in which the patients have been studied leave many questions about the nature and significance of the described changes.

V. WORK PERFORMANCE

Limitations in work performance have traditionally been attributed to the attendant anemia rather than to the metabolic consequences of iron deficiency. To Dr. Finch it seemed possible that a lesion in the muscle may exist but be obscured by the presence of anemia.[23] Indeed, recent experimental work in the rat indicates that a deficit in tissue iron is more important than anemia. A treadmill was used to measure the work performance of normal and iron-deficient rats. In iron-deficient rats, the initial running time was 4 min on day 0. There was a significant improvement in performance 1 d after iron administration, and the impairment in running ability was fully corrected within 4 d, indicating that the abnormalities imposed by iron deficiency are rapidly reversible (Figure 3). This was the effect of iron and not the correction of anemia — all groups were adjusted to a similar hemoglobin concentration by red cell transfusion.

It is not known whether these changes brought about by 4 d of iron therapy has a counterpart in man. However, in a recent report, the effect of 2 weeks of iron therapy on exercise performance and exercise-induced lactate production was measured in trained athletes. All the performance parameters measured on a bicycle ergometer were unchanged after iron therapy, but blood lactate levels at maximum exercise decreased significantly from 10.3 to 8.4 mM in the iron-deficient women following therapy ($p < 0.03$). These observations suggest that muscles call on anaerobic metabolism for energy needs with greater lactate production.[58] Another series of studies also suggests that the low hemoglobin level is not the major deficit in chronic iron deficiency.[15] When iron-deficient subjects were given an i.v. injection of iron dextran, work performance improved slightly more rapidly than the rise in hemoglobin, suggesting that iron had an effect not only related to relief of anemia. Further studies of work performance are needed to provide clear understanding of tissue iron deficiency and work performance in man.

VI. BEHAVIORAL ASPECTS

Whereas there has been a clinical impression of altered behavior (i.e., apathy, chronic fatigue, irritability, and a lack of interest in surroundings), and a widespread belief that these disturbances can be relieved promptly by the administration of iron before any significant rise in hemoglobin level, it has been difficult to demonstrate a clear relationship between iron deficiency and these effects. Clinical studies in children have been criticized

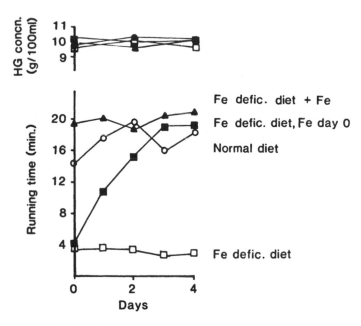

FIGURE 3.   Effect of iron therapy on running time on treadmill in four groups of rats. Hemoglobin levels in normal and iron-deficient animals were maintained at 10 g/dl.

as methodologically unsound, and studies in adults have given conflicting results.[3,43,59-61] Moreover, in many of the earlier studies, especially those in children, it has not been possible to distinguish the effects of iron deficiency from other factors, such as nutritional and social deprivation.[63] Also, tests to evaluate mental development in children are crude and in adults it has been difficult to differentiate the responders to iron from placebo effects.

Despite these limitations, the assessment of mental development and performance in normal and iron-deficient infants (0 to 2 years) by the Bayley Scales of Infant Development (BSID) showed impaired attention span and cognitive developmental abnormalities in the iron-deficient group with surprising consistency. Iron therapy (3 to 4 mg iron per kilogram per day) returned the mental development index (MDI) for iron-deficient infants to control values in 10 to 15 d and was without effect on the control infants. An improvement in cooperativeness and attention span on the BSID was also noted. A similar rapid improvement in cognitive function has also been reported by Oski and Honig.[61] However, other observations suggest that detectable abnormalities of neurological functions related to iron deficiency appear only in later infancy.[20,22]

In iron-deficient preschool children (3 to 6 years) a deficit in directing attention rather than a learning rate deficiency was observed.[59] Similarly, in iron-deficient school children (6 to 12), a deficit in directed attention with a secondary effect on scholastic achievement appeared to be the primary abnormality.

In adults clear evidence of an association between iron deficiency and psychological or cognitive function has not been obtained.[64] Chronic fatigue and other nonspecific symptoms were reported to respond to iron therapy in some individuals in some studies, but other investigators have produced conflicting results.[55] This illustrates the difficulty of establishing a relationship between iron deficiency and behavior, particularly when a variety of adverse environmental factors are also associated with iron deficiency.[44,62]

The rarity of nonhematological effects of iron deficiency has been noted in a recent study in adult patients with polycythemia vera who were treated exclusively with venesections for periods as long as 15 years.[51] The resulting chronic iron deficiency was manifested by microcytosis of the red cells, low serum iron, and reduced saturation of the iron-binding

TABLE 1
Biochemical Abnormalities Associated With Iron
Deficiency

Decrease in heme proteins
  Myoglobin
  Cytochromes
  Catalase
Decrease in activity of iron-containing enzymes
  Succinate dehydrogenase
  Monoamine oxidase
  α-Glycerophosphate oxidase
Decrease in activity of enzymes in which iron serves as cofactor
  Aconitase
Disturbed nucleic acid synthesis

protein. Some patients had chronic fatigue states believed to be related to depression. Administration of iron to one did not relieve fatigue but did cause rapid recurrence of polycythemia. Treadmill exercises were completed by six patients with results that indicated normal neuromuscular and cardiovascular function. None of the patients had dysphagia, glossitis, fissures at the corners of the mouth, or spoon-shaped nails. The only detectable nonhematologic manifestations of the chronic iron deficiency was pica, which consisted of compulsive ice eating and occurred more often in women than in men. These observations indicated that in persons of middle age or older, a degree of chronic iron deficiency sufficient to produce microcytosis of the red cells did not have serious untoward effects. Iron deficiency of a degree similar to that produced in the adult patients may have quite different effects on infants and children where, as mentioned before, decreased motivation, decreased attention span, and an overall impairment in intellectual performance has been described as well as a reduction in involuntary activity.

VII. BIOCHEMICAL ABNORMALITIES

Iron participates in a wide range of biochemical processes, such as mitochondrial electron transport, catecholamine metabolism, and DNA synthesis.[12,65-67] In iron deficiency, an overall reduction in the amount or in the activity of many iron-dependent enzymes or storage forms of iron has been reported (Table 1); however, there are differences between tissues and the degree to which they can protect essential iron. Factors that seem to favor the development of tissue iron deficiency include rapid tissue growth, rapid cell turnover, or both. For example, the maintenance of mitochondrial iron in the heart is better than in striated muscle.[12,23] Even within individual tissues in subcellular compartments some compounds are affected far more than others.[12,67] Thus, in the liver parenchymal cell, the mitochondrial cytochromes are more readily depleted than the cytochromes in the endoplasmic reticulum, and in the endoplasmic reticulum, cytochrome P450 is more affected than cytochrome B5.[12,65] Thus, an understanding of the physiologic effects becomes more complicated since they are both organ and compartment related. Furthermore, such biochemical changes have been observed in iron-deficient man in the presence of anemia, but also in its absence.[24]

Sometimes the significance of molecular abnormalities in iron deficiency is reflected in the structural and functional changes associated with them. There is an enlargement and electron lucency of mitochondria from liver and muscle of iron-deficient animals and of lymphocytes of iron-deficient men.[20] The impairment in proliferation of red cell precursors and the transformation of lymphocytes is paralleled by general impairment in DNA synthesis in experimental animals, perhaps due to inhibition of ribonucleotide reductase.[10,68]

A variety of effects due to deficiency of essential tissue iron has been demonstrated in animals. Fetal development in pregnant rats is retarded and stopped in the presence of maternal iron deficiency.[11] Muscle dysfunction has been found in iron-deficient adult animals when anemia has been corrected by exchange transfusion.[23] On exertion, these animals acquire a lactic acidosis that prevents further activity. Mitochondrial enzyme, α-glycerophosphate oxidase, appears to be responsible for the impaired cellular metabolism. Increased catecholamine levels have been described in iron-deficient children, and it has been suggested that behavioral abnormalities are associated with this deficiency of iron.[12,69,70] Other experimental work has shown impaired thermogenesis and impaired response to iodothyronine to cold in iron deficiency anemia.[12,69-72] In the intestinal mucosa, enzyme depletion of cytochrome P450 and cytochrome oxidase has been demonstrated, but there is no convincing evidence to link this to gastrointestinal symptoms and/or dysfunction.[66]

The underlying physiological mechanisms influencing behavior are largely speculative. Several parts of the brain contain large quantities of iron,[53,73] and iron is required for the activity of enzymes, such as tyrosine hydroxylase, tryptophane hydroxylase, and monoamine oxidase which are important to neurotransmitter metabolism. A series of studies in rats carried out by Youdim et al.[71] suggests that dopamine receptor function is impaired in iron deficiency and leads to the observed neurophysiological changes. More recent reports suggest that there is a neuropeptide-like distribution pattern of transferrin receptors in the brain.[74] This suggests that transferrin, in addition to transporting iron, may modulate behavior like other neuropeptides and lack of iron would interfere with this function.

In summary, the attribution of specific physical findings to tissue heme protein deficiency at this moment is largely speculative. However, it is likely that iron deficiency interferes with the overall oxidative metabolism in man.[69,70] Although our understanding of the consequences of tissue iron deficiency is undoubtedly fragmentary at this time, the studies discussed above provide ample reason for concern and a convincing rationale for programs to ensure adequate iron nutrition in the growing child.

REFERENCES

1. **Cook, J. D. and Lynch, S. R.,** The liabilities of iron deficiency, *Blood,* 68, 803, 1986.
2. **Charlton, R. W. and Bothwell, T. H.,** Definition, prevalence and prevention of iron deficiency, in *Clinics in Haematology,* 11th ed., W. B. Saunders, Philadelphia, 1982, 309.
3. **Pollitt, E. and Leibel, R. L.,** Iron deficiency and behavior, *J. Pediatr.,* 88, 372, 1976.
4. **Basta, S. S., Soekirman, M. S., Karyadi, D., et al.,** Iron deficiency anemia and the productivity of adult males in Indonesia, *J. Clin. Nutr.,* 32, 916, 1979.
5. **Gardner, G. W., Edgerton, V. R., Senewiratne, B., et al.,** Physical work capacity and metabolic stress in subjects with iron deficiency anemia, *Am. J. Clin. Nutr.,* 30, 910, 1977.
6. **Edgerton, V. R., Gardner, G. W., and Ohira, Y., et al.,** Iron-deficiency anaemia and its effect on worker productivity and activity patterns, *Br. Med. J.,* 2, 1546, 1979.
7. **Rasch, C. A., Cotton, E. K., Griggs, R. C., et al.,** Shortened survival of autotransfused 51Cr-labeled erythrocytes in infants with severe iron-deficiency anemia, *Semin. Hematol.,* 13, 181, 1976.
8. **Ohira, Y., Edgerton, V. R., and Gardner, G. W., et al.,** Serum lipid levels in iron deficiency anemia and effects of various treatments, *J. Nutr. Sci. Vitaminol.,* 26, 375, 1980.
9. **Bierman, E. L.,** Hyperlipemia and iron deficiency, *Nutr. Rev.,* 33, 55, 1975.
10. **Siimes, M. A. and Dallman, P. R.,** Iron deficiency: impaired liver growth and DNA synthesis in the rat, *Br. J. Haematol.,* 28, 453, 1974.
11. **Finch, C. A., Huebers, H. A., Miller, L., Josephson, B., Shepard, T., and Mackler, B.,** Fetal iron balance in the rat, *Am. J. Clin. Nutr.,* 37, 910, 1983.

12. **Beard, J., Finch, C. A., and Mackler, B.,** Deleterious effects of iron deficiency, in *Nutrition in Health and Disease and International Development: Symp. XII Int. Cong. Nutrition,* Alan R. Liss, New York, 1981, 305.
13. **Rothenbacher, H. and Sherman, A. R.,** Target organ pathology in iron-deficient suckling rats, *J. Nutr.,* 110, 1648, 1980.
14. **Prime, S. S., MacDonald, D. G., and Rennie, J. S.,** The effect of iron deficiency on experimental oral carcinogenesis in the rat, *Br. J. Cancer,* 47, 413, 1983.
15. **Finch, C. A., Beard, J. L., Huebers, H. A., et al.,** Tissue iron deficiency, in *Practical Approaches to Eradication of Subclinical Iron Deficiency,* Inoue and Suzue, Eds., Malnutrition Panel of U.S.-Japan Cooperative Medical Science Program, Tokyo, 1983.
16. **Finch, C. A. and Huebers, H.,** Perspective in iron metabolism, *N. Engl. J. Med.,* 306, 1520, 1982.
17. **Dallman, P. R.,** Manifestations of iron deficiency, *Semin. Hematol.,* 19, 19, 1982.
18. **Dallman, P. R., Beutler, E., and Finch, C. A.,** Annotation: effects of iron deficiency exclusive of anaemia, *Br. J. Haematol.,* 40, 179, 1978.
19. **Siimes, M. A., Refino, C., and Dallman, P. R.,** Manifestation of iron deficiency at various levels of dietary iron intake, *Am. J. Clin. Nutr.,* 33, 570, 1980.
20. **Leibel, R., Greenfield, D., and Pollitt, E.,** Annotation: Biochemical and behavioural aspects of sideropenia, *Br. J. Haematol.,* 41, 145, 1979.
21. **Finch, C. A., Miller, L. R., Inamdar, A. R., Person, R., Seiler, K., and Macker, B.,** Iron deficiency in the rat. Physiological and biochemical studies of muscle dysfunction, *J. Clin. Invest.,* 58, 447, 1976.
22. **Cook, J. D. and Lynch, S. R.,** The liabilities of iron deficiency, *Blood,* 447, 1986.
23. **Weinberg, E. D.,** Iron withholding: a defense against infection and neoplasia, *Physiol. Rev.,* 1, 65, 1984.
24. **Pollitt, E., Soemantri, A. G., Yunis, F., et al.,** Cognitive effects of iron-deficiency anaemia, *Lancet,* 1, 65, 1985.
25. **Krantman, H. J., Young, S. R., Ank, B. J., et al.,** Immune function in pure iron deficiency, *Am. J. Dis. Child.,* 136, 840, 1982.
26. **Hunter, R. L., Bennett, B., Towns, M., et al.,** Transferrin in disease. II. Defects in the regulation of transferrin saturation with iron contribute to susceptibility to infection, *Am. J. Clin. Pathol.,* 31, 748, 1984.
27. **Richter, G. W.,** Studies of iron overload, *Lab. Invest.,* 50, 26, 1984.
28. **Burman, D.,** Anaemia in infancy — is iron important?, *Proc. R. Soc. Med.,* 64, 579, 1971.
29. **Josephs, H. W.,** Hypochromic microcytic anemia of infancy: iron depletion as a factor, *Pediatrics,* 18, 959, 1956.
30. **Hillman, R. S. and Finch, C. A.,** *Red Cell Manual,* 5th ed., F.A. Davis, Philadelphia, 1985, 1.
31. **Dallman, P. R. and Siimes, M. A.,** Percentile curves for hemoglobin and red cell volume in infancy and childhood, *J. Pediatr.,* 94, 26, 1979.
32. **Cazzola, M., Heubers, H. A., Sayers, M. H., MacPhail, A. P., Eng, M., and Finch, C. A.,** Transferrin saturation, plasma iron turnover and transferrin uptake in normal humans, *Blood,* 66, 935, 1985.
33. **Finch, C. A. and Huebers, H. A.,** Iron metabolism, *Clin. Physiol. Biochem.,* 4, 5, 1986.
34. **Beard, J., Green, W., Miller, L., and Finch, C. A.,** Effect of anemia and iron deficiency on thermoregulation and thyroid hormone levels during cold exposure, *Am. J. Physiol.,* 247, R114, 1984.
35. **Labbe, R. F., Finch, C. A., Smith, M. J., et al.,** Erythrocyte protoporphyrin/heme ratio in the assessment of iron status, *Clin. Chem.,* 25, 87, 1979.
36. **Labbe, R. F. and Finch, C. A.,** Erythrocyte protoporphyrin: application in the diagnosis of iron deficiency, in *Iron,* Cook, J. D., eds., Churchill Livingston, New York, 1980, 44.
37. **English, E. C. and Finch, C. A.,** Iron deficiency: a systematic approach, *Drug Ther.,* 14, 45, 1984.
38. **Josephs, H. W.,** Iron metabolism and the hypochromic anemia of infancy, *Medicine,* 32, 125, 1953.
39. **Cook, J. D., Alvarado, J., Gutnisky, A., et al.,** Nutritional deficiency and anemia in Latin America: a collaborative study, *Blood,* 38, 591, 1971.
40. **MacKay, H. M.,** Anemia in infancy: its prevalence and prevention, *Arch. Dis. Child.,* 3, 117, 1928.
41. **Vyas, D. and Chandra, R. K.,** Functional implications of iron deficiency, in *Iron Nutrition in Infancy and Childhood,* Stekel, A., Ed., Raven Press, New York, 1984, 45.
42. **Cook, J. D. and Finch, C. A.,** Assessing iron status of a population, *Am. J. Clin. Nutr.,* 32, 2115, 1979.
43. **Burman, D.,** Hemoglobin levels in normal infants aged 3 to 24 months, and the effect of iron, *Arch. Dis. Child.,* 47, 261, 1972.
44. **Bernat, I.,** *Iron Deficiency in Iron Metabolism,* Plenum Press, New York, 1983, 215.
45. **Bernat, I.,** *Ozaena — A Manifestation of Iron Deficiency,* Pergamon Press, Oxford, 1965.
46. **Bernat, I.,** *Die Ozaena — eine Manifestation der Eisenmangelkrankheit,* Akademiaei Kiado, Budapest and VEB Verlag Volk, Berlin, 1966.
47. **Oski, F. A.,** The nonhematologic manifestations of iron deficiency, *Am. J. Dis. Child.,* 133, 315, 1979.
48. **Chisholm, M.,** The association between webs, iron and post-cricoid carcinoma, *Postgrad. Med. J.,* 50, 215, 1974.

49. **Rector, W. G., Jr., Fortuin, N. J., and Conley, C. L.**, Non-hematologic effects of chronic iron deficiency. A study of patients with polycythemia vera treated solely with venesections, *Medicine,* 61, 382, 1982.

50. **Witts, L. J.**, *Hypochromic Anaemia,* William Heinemann, London, 1969, 1.

51. **Bothwell, T. H., Charlton, R. W., Cook, J. D., and Finch, C. A.**, *Iron Metabolism in Man,* Blackwell Scientific, Oxford, 1979.

52. **Hardison, J. E.**, An ice crusher for Aunt Linna, *JAMA,* 249, 2769, 1983.

53. **Elwood, P. C. and Wood, M. M.**, Effect of oral iron therapy on the symptoms of anaemia, *Br. J. Prev. Soc. Med.,* 20, 172, 1966.

54. **Judisch, J. M., Naiman, J. L., and Oski, F. A.**, The fallacy of the fat iron-deficient child, *Pediatrics,* 37, 987, 1966.

55. **Badenoch, J., Evans, J. R., and Richards, W. C. D.**, The stomach in hypochromic anaemia, *Br. J. Haematol.,* 3, 175, 1957.

56. **Schoene, R. B., Escourrou, P., Robertson, H. T., et al.**, Iron depletion decreases maximal exercise lactate concentrations in female athletes with minimal iron-deficiency anemia, *J. Lab. Clin. Med.,* 102, 306, 1983.

57. **Pollitt, E., Leibel, R. L., Greenfield, D. B., and Greenfield, D. B.**, Iron deficiency and cognitive test performance in preschool children, *Nutr. Behav.,* 1, 137, 1983.

58. **Williams, R. A., Samson, D., Tikerpae, J., et al.**, *In-vitro* studies of ineffective erythropoiesis in rheumatoid arthritis, *Anal. Rheum. Dis.,* 41, 502, 1982.

59. **Soemantri, A. G., Pollitt, E., and Kim, I.**, Iron deficiency anemia and educational achievement, *Am. J. Clin. Nutr.,* 42, 1221, 1985.

60. **Weintraub, L. R., Conrad, M. E., and Crosby, W. H.**, The treatment of hemochromatosis by phlebotomy, *Med. Clin. North Am.,* 50, 1579, 1966.

61. **Oski, F. A. and Honig, A. S.**, The effect of therapy on the developmental scores of iron-deficiency infants, *J. Pediatr.,* 92, 21, 1978.

62. **Webb, T. E. and Oski, F. A.**, Behavioral status of young adolescents with iron deficiency anemia, *J. Spec. Educ.,* 8, 153, 1974.

63. **Bailey-Wood, R., Blayney, L. M., Muir, J. R., et al.**, The effects of iron deficiency on rat liver enzymes, *Br. J. Exp. Pathol.,* 56, 193, 1975.

64. **Dagg, J. H., Jackson, J. M., Curry, B., et al.**, Cytochrome oxidase in latent iron deficiency (sideropenia), *Br. J. Haematol.,* 12, 331, 1966.

65. **Mackler, B., Person, R., Ochs, H., and Finch, C. A.**, Iron deficiency in the rat: effects on neutrophil activation and metabolism, *Pediatr. Res.,* 18, 459, 1984.

66. **Kuvibidila, S., Nauss, K. M., Baliga, B. S., et al.**, Impairment of blastogenic response of splenic lymphocytes from iron-deficient mice: *in vivo* repletion, *Am. J. Clin. Nutr.,* 37, 15, 1983.

67. **Dillman, E., Mackler, B., Johnson, D., Brengelmann, G., Green, W., Gale, C., Martin, J., Layrisse, M., Martinez-Torres, C., and Finch, C. A.**, Effect of iron deficiency on catecholamine metabolism and body temperature regulation, in *Iron Deficiency: Brain Biochemistry and Behavior,* Pollitt, E. and Liebel, R. L., Eds. Raven Press, New York, 1982, 57.

68. **Mackler, B. and Finch, C.**, Iron in central nervous system oxidative metabolism, in *Iron Deficiency: Brain Biochemistry and Behaviour,* Pollitt, E. and Liebel, R. L., Eds., Raven Press, New York, 1982, 31.

69. **Dillman, E., Gale, C., Green, W., Johnson, D., Mackler, B., and Finch, C. A.**, Hypothermia in iron deficiency due to altered triiodothyronine metabolism, *Am. J. Physiol.,* 239, R377, 1980.

70. **Beard, J. L., Finch, C. A., and Green, W. L.**, Interactions of iron deficiency, anemia, and thyroid hormone levels in the response of rats to cold exposure, *Life Sci.,* 30, 691, 1982.

71. **Youdim, M. B. H., Yehuda, S., Ben-Schchar, D., and Askenazi, R.**, Behavioral and brain biochemical changes in iron-deficient rats: the involvement of iron in dopamine receptor function, in *Iron Deficiency: Brain Biochemistry and Behavior,* Pollitt, E. and Leibel, R. L., Eds., Raven Press, New York, 1982, 39.

72. **Hill, J. M., Ruff, M. R., Weber, R. J., and Pert, C. B.**, Transferrin receptors in rat brain: neuropeptide-like pattern and relationship to iron distribution, *Proc. Natl. Acad. Sci. U.S.A.,* 82, 4553, 1985.

Chapter 4

IRON, OXYGEN STRESS, AND THE PRETERM INFANT

Lennart T. Jansson

TABLE OF CONTENTS

"Having filled a vial with our Air (empyreal) I poured in some colourless animal oil and stopped it up very carefully; a few hours after it was become brown and the next day black."

C.W. Scheele, 1780

I. INTRODUCTION

The experiment cited above was performed over 200 years ago by C. W. Scheele.[1] He was one of the discoverers of oxygen (or empyreal air [fire air] as he called it). In the experiment with oxygen and animal oil he witnessed an oxidative decomposition of lipids. This finding illustrates that oxygen, although vital to aerobic life, also has toxic properties. The reactions and chemical species that mediate the toxic effects of oxygen have become recognized first during the last decades.

Oxygen in concentrations exceeding 21% is toxic to both plants and animals. These toxic effects are primarily caused by highly reactive products of oxygen: the oxygen derived radicals.[2-4] This chapter concerns the formation of oxygen radicals, the role of iron in the toxicity of oxygen, antioxidative protective mechanisms, and the clinical implications of oxygen toxicity for the preterm infant.

II. OXYGEN RADICALS

A. FREE RADICALS

A free radical is a chemical species (atom, group of atoms, or molecule) possessing one or more unpaired electrons. Oxygen has two unpaired electrons and is thus by definition a bi-radical (Table 1). Both these unpaired electrons of oxygen have the same spin quantum number. From this follows that if oxygen accepts a pair of electrons from another atom, both these electrons must be of parallel spin. This phenomenon, usually referred to as "spin restriction", diminishes the reactivity of oxygen because a pair of electrons in an atomic orbital would have antiparallel spins (Pauli's principle). Oxygen, therefore, tends to accept one electron at a time. The spin restriction of molecular oxygen is bypassed in the normal metabolic reduction of oxygen by the enzyme cytochrome oxidase. This enzyme contains heme iron at the active site that donates electrons to molecular oxygen without the release of the radicals. Oxygen not metabolized by cytochrome oxidase or another enzyme may, in the presence of an electron donor (for example, the transition metals copper or iron), be subjected to a one electron reduction and form a free radical (Table 1). The generation of these radicals may have important consequences in the process of cell aging in aerobic organisms.[5]

B. SUPEROXIDE RADICALS

A one-electron reduction of oxygen gives rise to the superoxide radical ($\cdot O_2^-$) (Table 1). $\cdot O_2^-$ is formed in almost all aerobic cells.[6] The generation of $\cdot O_2^-$ is associated with several deleterious effects on the organism including DNA degeneration,[4] loss of viscosity of human synovial fluid,[7] and damage to cell membranes.[8] The generation of $\cdot O_2^-$ is also a vital part in the bacterial killing by phagocytic cells. $\cdot O_2^-$ is released in neutrophils, eosinophils, monocytes, and macrophages in a series of metabolic events usually referred to as "respiratory burst". $\cdot O_2^-$, however, is by itself quite unreactive.[10] The toxic effects seen after the generation of $\cdot O_2^-$ are considered to be caused by the formation of more reactive oxidizing radicals, especially the hydroxyl radical.[11]

C. SINGLET OXYGEN

Singlet oxygen is formed if the spin of one of the unpaired electrons of oxygen is changed in a way that permits oxygen to react with a nonradical (Table 1). Singlet oxygen is, therefore, a very reactive species. Formation of singlet oxygen has been recognized if porphyrins are exposed to visible light[12] and in the lens and the retina of the mammalian eye.[13]

TABLE 1
Oxygen and Oxygen-Derived Radicals, Electron Configuration in Highest Occupied Orbitals

Oxygen (O_2)	↑	↑
Superoxide (O_2^-)	↑↓	↑
Singlet oxygen ($^1\Delta O_2$)	↑↓	
Singlet oxygen ($^1\Sigma g^+$)	↑	↓

Note: The arrows denote the direction of electron spin.

D. HYDROGEN PEROXIDE, HYDROXYL RADICAL, AND METAL CATALYSTS

Addition of another electron to $\cdot O_2^-$ yields the peroxide anion (O_2^-), which protonates rapidly to generate hydrogen peroxide (H_2O_2) (Equation 1).

$$2O_2^- + 2H^+ \rightarrow H_2O_2 + O_2 \qquad (1)$$

This reaction (Equation 1) is called the dismutation reaction and is catalyzed by the enzyme superoxide dismutase (SOD). H_2O_2 is toxic by itself, but becomes more so after reacting with $\cdot O_2^-$, resulting in formation of the hydroxyl radical (OH$\cdot$) (Equation 2).

$$\cdot O_2^- + H_2O_2 \rightarrow OH\cdot + OH^- + O_2 \qquad (2)$$

Reaction 2 is called the Haber-Weiss reaction[14] and occurs *in vitro* in the presence of iron (Equations 3 to 5).

$$\cdot O_2^- + Fe^{3+} \rightarrow O_2 + Fe^{2+} \qquad (3)$$

$$2O_2^- + 2H^+ \rightarrow H_2O_2 + O_2 \qquad (4)$$

$$Fe^{2+} + H_2O_2 \rightarrow Fe^{3+} + HO\cdot + HO^- \qquad (5)$$

In aqueous solution, iron exists in two oxidation states: ferrous (Fe^{2+}) and ferric (Fe^{3+}).[15] During the oxidation of Fe^{2+}, there is a possibility for a one electron reduction of oxygen; however, iron bound to proteins does not behave as a transition metal. Iron enters the cell bound to the protein transferrin. Intracellularly released iron probably chelates with other compounds, for example, citrate. The chelated iron is then used in the synthesis of iron proteins. The iron that is not used in the cell is stored as ferritin. Iron is taken up as Fe^{2+} by apoferritin and oxidized to Fe^{3+} before storage in the interior of the ferritin molecules. Thus, there exists intracellularly a small pool of chelated nonprotein bound iron that may participate in redox reactions. Whether these reactions occur *in vivo* is the subject of some debate,[16] as described in a recent review.[3]

The hydroxyl radical is a more reactive radical than $\cdot O_2^-$ and can, if formed *in vivo*, react with almost all types of organic molecules including the membrane lipids and intitiate lipid peroxidation.

E. LIPID PEROXIDATION

Peroxidation of membrane lipids can be initiated by an attack of a radical that is reactive enough to abstract a hydrogen atom (H) from an unsaturated fatty acid (LH) with the formation of a carbon radical (L$\cdot$) on the unsaturated fatty acid (Equation 6).

$$LH \rightarrow L\cdot + H^+ \tag{6}$$

This carbon radical stabilizes rapidly by a molecular rearrangement to form a conjugated diene that immediately reacts with oxygen forming a fatty acid peroxyl radical (LOO·) (Equation 7).

$$L\cdot + O_2 \rightarrow LOO\cdot \tag{7}$$

The peroxyl radical then abstracts hydrogen atoms from other lipid molecules and fatty acid hydroperoxides (LOOH) are formed (Equation 8).

$$LOO\cdot + LH \rightarrow LOOH + L\cdot \tag{8}$$

Decomposition of these hydroperoxides can be catalyzed by transition metals. Iron compounds react with lipid hydroperoxides to give alkoxy (Lipid-O·) and peroxy (Lipid-O$_2$·) radicals (Equations 9 to 10).[3]

$$\text{Lipid-OOH} + Fe^{2+}\text{-complex} \rightarrow Fe^{2+}\text{-complex} + OH^- + \text{Lipid-O}\cdot \tag{9}$$

$$\text{Lipid-OOH} + Fe^{3+}\text{-complex} \rightarrow \text{Lipid-OO}\cdot + H^+ + Fe^{2+}\text{-complex} \tag{10}$$

Both these radicals (lipid-O· and lipid-O$_2$·) can abstract more hydrogen atoms and further stimulate lipid peroxidation.

III. ANTIOXIDANT DEFENSE

Through the reactions related above, oxygen is a constant threat to life. During evolution, several mechanisms have evolved to protect aerobic organisms from attacks by oxygen-derived radicals. These protective mechanisms work through enzymatic factors, factors involving structural integrity, factors that diminish the availability of transition metals, and by free-radical scavengers, such as vitamin E.

A. PROTECTIVE MECHANISMS
1. Enzymatic

Three enzymes are known to participate in the protection against oxygen derived radicals: superoxide dismutase (SOD), glutathione-peroxidase (GSH-Px), and catalase (CAT). The actions of these enzymes are summarized in Equations 1 and 11 to 13.

SOD accelerates the dismutation reaction (Equation 1). The SOD enzymes remove formed ·O$_2^-$ and, therefore, prevent the formation of ·OH. Three forms of SOD exist in humans: copper-zinc SOD[17] is found in the cytoplasm and in the mitochondrial intermembrane space; manganese SOD[18] is found in the mitochondrial matrix. Recently, an extracellular SOD containing both copper and zinc was also described.[19] GSH-Px protects cellular and subcellular elements from oxidative injury. It is present in almost all mammalian cells.[20] Two forms exist: seleno- and nonseleno-GSH-Px. The seleno-GSH-Px catalyzes the reduction of hydrogen peroxide (H$_2$O$_2$) to water:

$$2GSH + H_2O_2 \xrightarrow{\text{GSH-Px}} GSSG + 2H_2O \tag{11}$$

The glutathione disulfide (GSSG) (oxidized glutathione) is then reconverted to reduced glutathione (GSH) by glutathione reductase (GR) (Equation 12).

$$GSSG + 2NADPH \xrightarrow{GR} 2GSH + 2NADP^+ \qquad (12)$$

The NADPH used in this reaction is generated via the hexose monophosphate shunt.

CAT, which is an iron containing enzyme, is found in the highest concentrations in erythrocytes and in liver tissue. The enzyme catalyzes the breakdown of H_2O_2 (Equation 13).

$$2H_2O_2 \xrightarrow{CAT} 2H_2O + O_2 \qquad (13)$$

2. Structural Integrity

Disruption of a tissue rapidly leads to rancidification through the propagation of lipid peroxidation reactions.[21,22] Loss of structural integrity can occur through either the disruption of whole cells or of subcellular elements. Therefore, structural integrity is of importance to minimize oxidant injury even at the molecular level.

Human plasma is a powerful antioxidant.[22] The major responsible factors are transferrin and ceruloplasmin. Both of these plasma products act by minimizing the availability of iron for participation in free-radical reactions. Ceruloplasmin is a ferroxidase[23] promoting the oxidation of ferrous iron (Fe^{2+}) to the ferric form (Fe^{3+}), thereby preventing iron from donating electrons to oxygen. In addition, ceruloplasmin may even directly scavenge the $\cdot O_2^-$ radical.[24] Transferrin is the iron transport protein in plasma. In healthy individuals, transferrin is not fully saturated with iron. This leaves a capacity to bind ionic iron in plasma. In patients with iron overload, transferrin may be fully saturated with iron, and there is evidence that some toxic effects of iron overload are caused by free-radical reactions.[25]

3. Free-Radical Scavengers

Another important system that protects the organism against attack by free radicals is that mediated by free-radical scavengers (AH). These molecules can directly scavenge a free radical ($L\cdot$) by donating a hydrogen atom to the radical, resulting in the formation of a scavenger radical ($A\cdot$) (Equation 14)

$$L\cdot + AH \rightarrow LH + A\cdot \qquad (14)$$

The most important free radical scavenger *in vivo* is vitamin E.[26] The scavenger radical ($A\cdot$) formed after the reaction between a lipid peroxide radical ($L\cdot$) and vitamin E is unreactive and degrades without injury to the organism. Vitamin E includes several different substances (isomers of tocopherol and tocotrienol). These all have antioxidant activity, but α-tocopherol is the most potent.[27] One site of action of vitamin E is in the hydrophobic interior of biological membranes.[28] An important function of vitamin E in biological membranes is to scavenge radicals formed in lipid peroxidation reactions.[29] In addition, vitamin E may also reduce superoxide anions and singlet oxygen.[30]

IV. OXYGEN TOXICITY AND THE NEONATE

A. OXYGEN TOXICITY

During intrauterine life, oxygen delivery via the placenta ensures a fetal arterial oxygen tension (pO_2) of 20 to 35 torr.[31] At birth, the newborn infant is exposed to the 21% environmental oxygen tension and the arterial pO_2 during the first hour of life is raised to about 50 to 60 torr.[32] This increase in pO_2 is accompanied by a 50% increase in O_2 consumption.[33] The rapid change from a relatively hypoxic to a relatively hyperoxic environment, in addition to an increase in the amount of oxygen that is metabolized, will increase the risk of oxygen-mediated toxicity in the infant. Indirect evidence also exists that this increased load of oxygen may have untoward effects on the newborn infant. In a recent study, Wispe et al.[34] found higher levels of ethane and pentane in the expired air from newborn infants compared to adults. Ethane and pentane are derived from the peroxidative decomposition of linolenic and linoleic acid. Therefore, the amounts of these compounds in expired air will be an indirect measure of the *in vivo* peroxidative degradation of those fatty acids.[35,36] A possible cause of an increased peroxidation of lipids in the newborn infant is an incomplete development of oxygen defense mechanisms.

During gestation, several mechanisms develop that have the function of preparing the newborn organism for the relatively high oxygen, postpartum milieu. These antioxidant mechanisms include enzymatic factors, factors related to molecular integrity, and to direct scavenging of oxygen-derived radicals. In the preterm infant, there is a delayed maturation of some of these defense mechanisms, which may render the preterm infant especially sensitive to the changes in oxygen milieu immediately after birth. In addition, supplemental oxygen often has to be given to preterm infants because of lung disease, which will further increase the oxygen load. Dietary interventions, such as iron treatment and supplementation with polyunsaturated fatty acids may also increase the susceptibility to oxygen radicals. Therefore, immaturity, supplemental oxygen, and dietary factors are the main factors that determine the occurrence of oxygen toxicity in preterm infants. Organs in which a disease state caused by oxygen-derived free radicals can develop are the lung, the eye, and the red blood cell.

B. OXYGEN TOXICITY AND LUNG DISEASE

Exposure of the human lung to high concentrations of oxygen will induce pathologic changes. These changes are characterized by an acute phase consisting of edema, hemorrhage, exudate, and necrosis of endothelial and type 1 alveolar cells.[37] After the acute phase, chronic changes occur including proliferation of type 2 alveolar cells, fibrosis, and deposition of collagen.[37] The main determinant of this oxygen toxicity supported by experimental evidence is the oxygen-tension in the alveolar lining.[38-40] The first cell type to be damaged, however, is the endothelial cell. This finding indicates that the oxygen tension inside the alveolar blood vessels also may be of importance in respect to oxygen toxicity in the lung. An explanation for this may be the release of oxygen-derived radicals from phagocytic cells.[41]

The pathologic lung changes occurring in preterm infants treated with supplemental oxygen, intubation, and positive pressure ventilation is called bronchopulmonary dysplasia (BPD).[42] BPD occurs in 11 to 21% of infants with hyaline membrane disease treated in this manner.[43] In addition to the high incidence of BPD in infants with hyaline membrane disease, it may also occur in similarly treated infants with congenital heart disease or other lung disease. Thus at least four important etiologic factors exist in the development of BPD: oxygen, intubation, immaturity, and pressure.

Prevention of BPD has been directed toward decreasing the use of high pressure in the ventilator, diminishing the time spent in the ventilator, and reducing the level of oxygen supplementation. Another mode of prevention that has also been tried is to increase the capacity of the organism to detoxify the oxygen-derived radicals with antioxidant enzymes and with the free radical scavenger, vitamin E.

C. ANTIOXIDANT ENZYMES AND BPD

The newborn mammal is more resistant to the acute toxic effects of oxygen than the adult animal. Experiments with newborn rats showed a survival rate of 100% after 120 h in 95% oxygen compared to about 20% survival of adult rats.[44,45] This finding can be attributed to the compensatory increases in lung antioxidant enzymes (SOD, GSH-Px, and

CAT) in neonatal animals.[37-44] Also, the level of pulmonary glutathione may increase in response to hyperoxia.[46] The pulmonary antioxidant enzyme level may, therefore, be an important factor in the development of lung disease secondary to hyperoxia.

During the maturation of the fetal mammalian lung, there is a continuous increase in the activity of enzymes that function in the detoxification of oxygen-derived radicals. Frank and Groseclose,[47] when measuring SOD, CAT, and GSH-Px in the fetal rabbit lung, found a significant increase in all these enzymes during the final days *in utero*. In the rat fetus, it was also possible to enhance the maturation of SOD, CAT, and GSH-Px by prenatal administration of dexamethasone.[48] This increase in antioxidant enzymes occurred simultaneously with the increase in lung surfactant.

The clinical implications of these animal experiments to humans are still not clear. Little is known about the antioxidant enzyme level in the lung of the human fetus. A single study by Autor et al.[49] demonstrated that lung tissue from six human fetuses aged 18 to 20 weeks contained a mean SOD content of 17 U/mg DNA compared to 370 U/mg DNA in preterm infants and 110 U/mg DNA in adults. A clinical trial studying the efficacy of bovine SOD given to preterm infants has also been conducted.[50] Experimental evidence, however, indicates that bovine SOD administered parenterally to rats does not penetrate the lung cells,[51] unless the SOD is encapsulated in liposomes.[52] Another, still experimental approach to increase lung antioxidant enzyme levels is by giving injections of endotoxin.[53]

D. VITAMIN E AND BPD

That the newborn preterm infant has low serum levels of vitamin E has long been recognized.[54] These low serum vitamin E levels have been claimed to be a result of a low transport capacity for vitamin E in these infants and not a sign of vitamin E deficiency.[55] The low serum vitamin E levels, however, are also associated with an increased sensitivity of the red blood cells to H_2O_2.[56] The increase in red cell H_2O_2 hemolysis and the observation that the increased H_2O_2 hemolysis is corrected by vitamin E supplementation, suggest that a true deficiency state may exist.[57]

Vitamin E deficiency in the laboratory animal increases oxygen toxicity to the lung.[58] In humans, two clinical trials have been performed to study the effects of supplemental vitamin E on the incidence of BPD in preterm infants with hyaline membrane disease. In the first preliminary study, a decreased incidence of BPD was seen following supplementation with pharmacologic doses of vitamin E.[59] This effect of vitamin E was, however, not reproduced in the follow-up study.[60] The treatment given to the infants differed between the two studies. During the first study,[59] higher pressures were used in the ventilators compared to the second study.[60] The etiology of BPD is multifactorial, and it is still a possibility that vitamin E administration may influence the development of BPD under certain conditions.

E. OXYGEN TOXICITY AND EYE DISEASE

The developing retina can be damaged when a preterm infant is exposed to prolonged hyperoxia. The infant is at risk of developing retrolental fibroplasia (RLF).[61] The pathologic changes in the retina caused by hyperoxia are characterized by vasospasm,[62] followed by necrosis of endothelial cells and proliferative changes.[63] The necrosis and the proliferation may be secondary to hypoxia.

RLF was originally seen in infants treated with oxygen,[61] and the incidence of the disease rapidly decreased when the use of oxygen diminished. The incidence of RLF, however, has increased again during the last decade. Factors other than oxygen that are important for the development of RLF are immaturity, intraventricular hemorrhage, bradycardia, septicemia, and acidosis.[64] RLF can also develop in immature infants not receiving supplemental oxygen.[65] It is, therefore, clear that the most judicious use of oxygen ensuring an arterial pO_2 not exceeding 50 to 60 torr, does not totally prevent the occurrence of RLF. Whether even the normal increase of arterial oxygen tension after birth can cause RLF is not known.

Studies on RLF in experimental animals have been unrewarding because of the lack of a suitable model. The retinopathy seen in kittens after exposure to hyperoxia does not progress to cicatricial retinal changes. In the kitten model, vitamin E reduces the oxygen toxicity to the retina.[66] One approach to preventing RLF has, therefore, been to increase the tissue resistance to oxygen radicals by supplementing the infants with vitamin E.

F. VITAMIN E AND RLF

The effect on the incidence of RLF by vitamin E supplementation to preterm infants has been studied by several investigators beginning with Owens and Owens in 1949.[67] In a large trial, Hittner et al.[68] found that a high oral dose of vitamin E (100 mg/kg/d) reduced both the incidence and severity of RLF in preterm infants with birthweights <1500 g. Finer et al.[69] who used i.m. vitamin E, also found a decreased severity of RLF in treated infants compared to controls, but a recent study by Phelps et al.[70] showed no effect on either incidence or severity of RLF by pharmacologic doses of vitamin E. The latter study, however, showed an increased incidence of intraventricular hemorrhage in the infants treated parenterally with vitamin E. This discrepancy with earlier investigations may be due to methodological differences, but the multifactorial etiology of RLF may also be of importance. Oxygen is only one of several factors predisposing to the development of RLF.

In the recent studies,[68-70] pharmacological doses of vitamin E were used, increasing serum vitamin E levels far above the levels found in healthy term infants. Possible negative effects of this could be a too effective scavenging of oxygen radicals, thus interfering with physiological metabolic events, such as the killing of bacteria by phagocytic cells. Clinical evidence now exists showing that vitamin E supplementation with high doses may be dangerous. A recent study showed a high incidence of both sepsis and necrotizing enterocolitis in vitamin E treated preterm infants.[71] Vitamin E in that study was given both parenterally and orally in order to achieve a serum level of 5 mg/dl.

V. NUTRITION AND OXYGEN STRESS

The nutritional status of a mammal may modify the toxic effects of oxygen by modulating antioxidant defense mechanisms. Nutrients that are of importance in this context are trace elements (as integral parts of antioxidant enzymes) and vitamin E (as an antioxidant in biological membranes). In addition, there are also nutrients that can increase oxidant stress, such as iron and polyunsaturated fatty acids (PUFA). In man, the association between dietary factors and oxygen toxicity is especially evident in the preterm infant. Nutrients proven to influence resistance to oxygen stress in preterm infants are iron, vitamin E, and PUFA, as an inappropriate supply of these nutrients may increase red cell hemolysis.

A. VITAMIN E

In the newborn infant, the plasma level of vitamin E is about one fifth that in the mother.[72] If the infant is fed a formula low in vitamin E, the low vitamin E levels may persist for several weeks in term infants and even decrease in infants born preterm.[72] The decrease in plasma vitamin E levels after birth is most pronounced in the smallest immature infants with birthweights below 1500 g.[73] This postnatal decrease in serum vitamin E levels may be caused both by smaller vitamin E stores at birth[74] and impaired intestinal absorption of vitamin E.[75] In small preterm infants, deficiency of vitamin E may cause increased red cell hemolysis. Oski and Barness[76] described preterm infants with hemolytic anemia and low serum vitamin E levels in whom vitamin E supplementation corrected the abnormality. A prospective study by the same authors[76] showed that a group of preterm infants given supplemental vitamin E had higher mean hemoglobin (Hb)-level compared to a control group. Subsequently this result has been confirmed by some investigators,[73,77-79] but not by others,[80-82] as summarized in recent reviews.[83,84] These discrepant results may be due to methodological differences, but may also be secondary to a different supply of other dietary factors that influence the vitamin E requirements. The most important dietary factors determining the vitamin E requirements are iron and PUFA.

B. IRON

Symptoms caused by vitamin E deficiency in experimental animals can be aggravated if iron is given.[85,86] This phenomenon is presumably caused by increased formation of toxic radicals generated in the reduction of oxygen.

Negative effects of the combination of vitamin E deficiency and treatment with iron can also develop in preterm infants. Melhorn and Gross[73] found lower Hb-levels in 6- to 10-week-old preterm infants when large doses of iron were given (8 to 10 mg/kg/d) compared to a large control group also given vitamin E supplementation. The negative effect on the Hb-level was most pronounced in the smallest infants (birthweights <1500 g). No negative effects of iron treatment were seen in the infants with birthweights >2000 g. These observations were ascribed to free radical-mediated hemolysis caused by vitamin E deficiency. Whether the red cell sensitivity to oxidant stress in preterm infants also is caused by a defect in the red blood cell antioxidant enzymes is not clear. Studies measuring SOD levels in red blood cells from preterm infants have shown both normal[49] and decreased[87] red cell SOD levels. In the studies by Melhorn and Gross,[73] a high level of supplemental iron was used (8 to 10 mg/kg/d); however, even a moderate dose of supplemental iron may cause hemolysis. Williams et al.[77] have shown that a supplement of 12 mg iron per liter formula (which makes about 2 mg/kg/d) increased red cell hemolysis in infants given a formula high in PUFA.

C. PUFA

The relationship between the dietary intake of PUFA and vitamin E and the oxidant injury to the newborn was investigated by Hassan et al.[88] They found that preterm infants fed a formula with 50% of the fatty acids as linoleic acid developed edema, skin lesions, elevated platelet count, and morphologic red cell changes. These abnormalities disappeared if vitamin E was given. Also, a more moderate increase in the intake of linoleic acid to about 30% of the total fatty acids may increase red cell hemolysis if supplemental iron is given.[77] In order to minimize such negative effects of the dietary PUFA, recommendations regarding the intake of PUFA and vitamin E also include a recommended vitamin E/PUFA ratio. According to the American Academy of Pediatrics, 1 IU of vitamin E should accompany each gram of linoleic acid fed to preterm infants.[89] In human milk, the vitamin E/PUFA ratio varies during lactation. In a study of milk from Swedish mothers, Jansson et al.[90] found mean α-tocopherol equivalent/linoleic acid ratios (mg/g) of 6.23 in colostrum, 1.43 in transitional milk, and 0.78 in mature milk. The preterm infant fed banked human milk that consists primarily of mature milk may, therefore, need an extra supplement of vitamin E. Even if the preterm infant is fed the mother's own breast milk (preterm milk), a daily supplement of vitamin E may be necessary.[91]

VI. CONCLUSIONS

Free radicals are formed during the reduction of oxygen. These oxygen-derived radicals are highly toxic to all kinds of animal cells. In the process of free-radical formation, iron is an important electron donor. Antioxidant enzymes and free-radical scavengers can quench free radicals formed in vivo.

The preterm infant has insufficient protection against free radicals because of immature defense mechanisms. This makes preterm infants especially sensitive to oxygen toxicity. Diseases in preterm infants now generally considered to be caused by the generation of oxygen-derived radicals are RLF, BPD, and oxidative hemolysis of red blood cells. Therapeutic interventions increasing the antioxidant protective capacity in preterm infants have been unsuccessful in reducing the incidence of RLF and BPD. The oxidative hemolysis in preterm infants can be prevented by regulating the dietary intake of iron, vitamin E, and PUFA.

REFERENCES

1. **Scheele, C. W.,** *Treatise on Air and Fire,* London, 1780.
2. **Del Maestro, R. F.,** An approach to free radicals in medicine and biology, *Acta Physiol. Scand.,* 492, 153, 1980.
3. **Halliwell, B. and Gutteridge, J. M. C.,** Oxygen toxicity, oxygen radicals, transition metals and disease, *Biochem. J.,* 219, 1, 1984.
4. **Halliwell, B.,** Oxygen is poisonous: the nature and medical importance of oxygen radicals, *Med. Lab. Sci.,* 41, 157, 1984.
5. **Pryor, W. A.,** Free radicals in autooxidation and aging, in *Free Radicals in Molecular Biology, Aging and Disease,* Armstrong, D., et al., Eds., Raven Press, New York, 1984, 13.
6. **Fridovich, I.,** The biology of oxygen radicals, *Science,* 201, 875, 1978.
7. **McCord, J. M.,** Free radicals and inflammation: protection of synovial fluid by superoxide dismutase, *Science,* 185, 529, 1974.
8. **Niehaus, W. G.,** A proposed role of superoxide anion as a biological nucleophile in the deesterification of phospholipids, *Bioorg. Chem.,* 7, 77, 1978.
9. **Babior, B. M.,** Oxidants from phagocytes: agents of defence and destruction, *Blood,* 64, 959, 1984.
10. **Halliwell, B.,** Superoxide-dependent formation of hydroxyl radicals in the presence of iron salts is a feasible source of hydroxyl radicals *in vivo, Biochem. J.,* 205, 461, 1982.
11. **Rosen, H. and Klebanoff, S. J.,** Hydroxyl radical generation by polymorphonuclear leucocytes measured by electron spin resonance spectroscopy, *J. Clin. Invest.,* 64, 1725, 1979.
12. **Foote, C. S.,** Light, oxygen and toxicity, in *Pathology of Oxygen,* Autor, A. P., Ed., Academic Press, New York, 1982, 21.
13. **Zigler, J. S. and Goosey, J. D.,** Photosensitized oxidation in the ocular lens: evidence for photosensitizers endogenous to the human lens, *Photochem. Photobiol.,* 33, 869, 1981.
14. **Haber, F. and Weiss, J.,** The catalytic decomposition of hydrogen peroxide by iron salts, *Proc. R. Soc. London Ser. A,* 147, 332, 1934.
15. **Aisen, P.,** Some physiochemical aspects of iron metabolism, in *Iron Metabolism,* Ciba Foundation Symp. 51, Elsevier/Exerpta Medica/North Holland, Amsterdam, 1977, 1.
16. **Winterbourn, C. C.,** Hydroxyl radical production in body fluids, roles of metal ions, ascorbate and superoxide, *Biochem. J.,* 198, 125, 1981.
17. **McCord, J. M. and Fridovich, I.,** Superoxide dismutase — an enzymatic function for erythrocuprein, *J. Biol. Chem.,* 244, 6049, 1969.
18. **Weisiger, R. A. and Fridovich, I.,** Mitochondrial superoxide dismutase. Site of synthesis and intramitochondrial localization, *J. Biol. Chem.,* 248, 4793, 1973.
19. **Marklund, S. L.,** Human copper-containing superoxide dismutase of high molecular weight, *Proc. Natl. Acad. Sci. U.S.A.,* 79, 7634, 1982.
20. **Sunde, R. A. and Hoekstra, W. G.,** Structure, synthesis and function of glutathione peroxidase, *Nutr. Rev.,* 38, 265, 1980.
21. **Willson, R. L.,** Iron, zinc, free radicals and oxygen in tissue disorders and cancer control, in *Iron Metabolism,* Ciba Found. Symp. 51, Elsevier/Exerpta Medica/North Holland, Amsterdam, 1977, 331.
22. **Dormandy, T. L.,** Free radical oxidation and antioxidants, *Lancet,* 1, 647, 1978.
23. **Osaki, S., Johnson, D. A., and Friedman, E.,** The possible significance of the ferrous oxidase activity of ceruloplasmin in normal human serum, *J. Biol. Chem.,* 241, 2746, 1966.
24. **Goldstein, I. M., Kaplan, H. B., Edelson, H. S., and Weissman, G.,** Ceruloplasmin: an acute phase reactant that scavenges oxygen-derived free radicals, *Ann. N.Y. Acad. Sci.,* 389, 368, 1982.
25. **Bacon, B. R., Tavill, A. S., Brittenham, G. M., Park, C. H., and Recknagel, R. O.,** Hepatic lipid peroxidation *in vivo* in rats with chronic iron overload, *J. Clin. Invest.,* 71, 429, 1983.

26. **McCay, P. B., Pfeifer, P. M., and Stipe, W. H.,** Vitamin E protection of membrane lipids during electron transport function, *Ann. N.Y. Acad. Sci.,* 203, 62, 1972.

27. **Horwitt, M. K.,** Vitamin E: a reexamination, *Am. J. Clin. Nutr.,* 29, 569, 1976.

28. **Lucey, J. A.,** Functional and structural aspects of biological membranes: a suggested structural role of vitamin E in the control of membrane permeability and stability, *Ann. N.Y. Acad. Sci.,* 203, 4, 1972.

29. **Tappel, A. L.,** Lipid peroxidation damage to cell components, *Fed. Proc.,* 32, 1870, 1973.

30. **Freeman, B. A. and Crapo, J. D.,** Biology of disease, free radicals and tissue injury, *Lab. Invest.,* 47, 412, 1982.

31. **Rudolph, A. M.,** The changes in the circulation after birth. Their importance in congenital heart disease, *Circulation,* 16, 343, 1970.

32. **Koch, G. and Wendel, H.,** Adjustment of arterial blood gases and acid-base balance in the normal newborn infant during the first week of life, *Biol. Neonat.,* 12, 136, 1968.

33. **Dawes, G. S. and Mott, J. C.,** The increase in oxygen consumption of the lamb after birth, *J. Physiol.,* 146, 295, 1959.

34. **Wispe, J. R., Bell, E. F., and Roberts, R. J.,** Assessment of lipid peroxidation in newborn infants and rabbits by measurements of expired ethane and pentane: influence of parenteral lipid infusion, *Pediatr. Res.,* 19, 374, 1985.

35. **Riely, C. A., Cohen, G., and Lieberman, M.,** Ethane evolution: a new index of lipid peroxidation, *Science,* 183, 208, 1974.

36. **Dillard, C. J., Dumelin, E. E., and Tappel, A. L.,** Effects of dietary vitamin E on expiration of pentane and ethane by the rat, *Lipids,* 12, 109, 1977.

37. **Frank, L.,** Effects of oxygen on the newborn, *Fed. Proc.,* 44, 2328, 1985.

38. **Wolfe, W. G., Ebert, P. A., and Sabiston, D. C.,** Effect of high oxygen tension on mucociliary function, *Surgery,* 72, 246, 1972.

39. **Ashbaugh, D. G.,** Oxygen toxicity in normal and hypoxemic dogs, *J. Appl. Physiol.,* 31, 664, 1971.

40. **Jentzen, J., Rockswold, G., and Anderson, W. R.,** Pulmonary oxygen toxic effect: occurrence in a newborn infant despite low PaO_2 due to an intracranial arteriovenous malformation, *Arch. Pathol. Lab. Med.,* 108, 334, 1984.

41. **Sacks, T., Moldow, C. F., Craddock, P. R., Bowers, T. K., and Jacob, H. S.,** Oxygen radicals mediate endothelial cell damage by complement stimulated granulocytes, *J. Clin. Invest.,* 61, 1161, 1978.

42. **Northaway, W. H., Jr., Rosan, R. C., and Porter, D. Y.,** Pulmonary disease following respiratory therapy of hyaline membrane disease: bronchopulmonary dysplasia, *N. Engl. J. Med.,* 276, 357, 1968.

43. **Northaway, W. H.,** Observations on bronchopulmonary dysplasia, *J. Pediatr.,* 95, 815, 1979.

44 **Yam, J., Frank, L., and Roberts, R. J.,** Oxygen toxicity: comparison of lung biochemical responses in neonatal and adult rats, *Pediatr. Res.,* 12, 115, 1978.

45. **Frank, L., Bucher, J. R., and Roberts, R. J.,** Oxygen toxicity in neonatal animals of various species, *J. Appl. Physiol.,* 45, 699, 1979.

46. **Warshaw, J. B., Wilson, C. W., Saito, S., and Russel, A. P.,** The responses of glutathione and antioxidant enzymes to hyperoxia in developing lung, *Pediatr. Res.,* 19, 819, 1975.

47. **Frank, L. and Groseclose, E. E.,** Preparation for birth into an O_2-rich environment: the antioxidant enzymes in the developing rabbit lung, *Pediatr. Res.,* 18, 240, 1984.

48. **Frank, L., Lewis, P. L., and Sosenko, I. R. S.,** Dexamethasone stimulation of fetal rat lung antioxidant enzyme activity in parallel with surfactant stimulation, *Pediatrics,* 75, 569, 1985.

49. **Autor, A. P., Frank, L., and Roberts, R. J.,** Developmental characteristics of pulmonary superoxide dismutase: relationship to idiopathic respiratory distress syndrome, *Pediatr. Res.,* 10, 154, 1976.

50. **Rosenfeld, W., Evans, H., Conception, L., Ihaveri, R., Schaeffer, H., and Friedman, A.,** Prevention of bronchopulmonary dysplasia by administration of bovine superoxide dismutase in preterm infants with respiratory distress syndrome, *J. Pediatr.,* 105, 781, 1984.

51. **Michelson, A. M. and Puget, K.,** Cell penetration by exogenous superoxide dismutase, *Acta Physiol. Scand. Suppl.,* 492, 67, 1980.

52. **Turrens, J. F., Crapo, J. D., and Freeman, B. A.,** Protection against oxygen toxicity by intravenous injection of liposome-entrapped catalase and superoxide dismutase, *J. Clin. Invest.,* 73, 87, 1984.

53. **Frank, L., Summerville, J., and Massaro, D.,** Protection from oxygen toxicity with endotoxin: role of the endogenous antioxidant enzymes of the lung, *J. Clin. Invest.,* 65, 1104, 1980.

54. **Bieri, J. G. and Farrell, P. M.,** Vitamin E, a reexamination, *Vitam. Horm.,* 34, 31, 1976.

55. **Hågå, P. and Kran, S.,** Plasma vitamin E levels and vitamin E/β-lipoprotein relationships in small preterm infants during the early anemia of prematurity, *Eur. J. Pediatr.,* 136, 143, 1981.

56. **Rose, C. S. and György, P.,** Specificity of hemolytic reaction in vitamin E-deficient erythrocytes, *Am. J. Physiol.,* 168, 414, 1952.

57. **Gutcher, G. R., Raynor, W. J., and Farrell, P. M.,** An evaluation of vitamin E status in premature infants, *Am. J. Clin. Nutr.,* 40, 1078, 1984.

58. **Wender, D. F., Thulin, G. E., Smith, G. J. W., and Warshaw, J. B.,** Vitamin E affects lung biochemical and morphologic response to hyperoxia in the newborn rabbit, *Pediatr. Res.,* 15, 262, 1981.

59. **Ehrenkranz, R. A., Bonta, B. W., Ablow, R. C., and Warshaw, J. B.,** Amelioration of bronchopulmonary dysplasia following vitamin E administration: a preliminary report, *N. Engl. J. Med.,* 299, 564, 1978.

60. **Ehrenkranz, R. A., Ablow, R. C., and Warshaw, J. B.,** Prevention of bronchopulmonary dysplasia with vitamin E administration during the acute stages of respiratory distress syndrome, *J. Pediatr.,* 95, 873, 1979.

61. **Kinsey, V. E.,** Retrolental fibroplasia: cooperative study of retrolental fibroplasia and the use of oxygen, *Arch. Ophthalmol.,* 56, 481, 1956.

62. **Nichols, C. W. and Lambertsen, C. J.,** Effects of high oxygen pressures on the eye, *N. Engl. J. Med.,* 281, 25, 1969.

63. **Foos, R. Y.,** Acute retrolental fibroplasia, *Albrecht von Graefes Arch. Klin. Exp. Ophthalmol.,* 195, 87, 1975.

64. **Lucey, J. F. and Dangman, B.,** A reexamination of the role of oxygen in retrolental fibroplasia, *Pediatrics,* 73, 82, 1984.

65. **Brockhurst, R. J. and Chishti, R. J.,** Cicatricial retrolental fibroplasia: its occurrence with oxygen administration and in full term infants, *Albrecht von Graefes Arch. Klin. Exp. Ophthalmol.,* 195, 113, 1975.

66. **Phelps, D. L. and Rosenbaum, A. L.,** The role of tocopherol in oxygen induced retinopathy: kitten model, *Pediatrics,* 59, 998, 1977.

67. **Owens, W. C. and Owens, E. V.,** Retrolental fibroplasia in premature infants: II. Studies on the prophylaxis of the disease: the use of alpha tocopherol acetate, *Am. J. Ophthalmol.,* 32, 1631, 1949.

68. **Hittner, H. M., Godio, L. B., Rudolph, A. J., Adams, J. M., Garcia-Prats, J. A., Friedman, Z., Kautz, J. A., and Monaco, W. A.,** Retrolental fibroplasia: efficacy of vitamin E in a double-blind clinical study of preterm infants, *N. Engl. J. Med.,* 305, 1365, 1981.

69. **Finer, N. N., Schindler, R. F., Grant, G., Hill, G. B., and Peters, K. L.,** Effect of intramuscular vitamin E on frequency and severity of retrolental fibroplasia. A controlled trial, *Lancet,* 1987, 1982.

70. **Phelps, D. L., Rosenbaum, A., Isenberg, S. J., Leake, R. D., and Dorey, F.,** Effect of iv tocopherol (vitamin E) on retinopathy of prematurity (ROP), *Pediatr. Res.,* 9, 357A, 1985.

71. **Johnson, L., Bowen, F. W., Abbasi, S., Herrmann, N., Weston, M., Sacks, L., Porat, R., Stahl, G., Peckham, G., Dellvora-Papadopoulos, M., Quinn, G., and Schaffer, D.,** Relationship of prolonged pharmacologic serum levels of vitamin E to increase of sepsis and necrotizing enterocolitis in infants with birth weight 1,500 grams or less, *Pediatrics,* 75, 619, 1985.

72. **Wright, S. W., Filer, L. J., Jr., and Mason, K. E.,** Vitamin E blood levels in premature and full term infants, *Pediatrics,* 7, 386, 1951.

73. **Melhorn, D. K. and Gross, S.,** Vitamin E dependent anemia in the premature infant. I. Effects of large doses of medicinal iron, *J. Pediatr.,* 79, 569, 1971.

74. **Dju, M. Y., Mason, K. E., and Filer, L. J., Jr.,** Vitamin E (tocopherol) in human fetuses and placenta, *Etudes Neo-Natales,* 1, 49, 1952.

75. **Melhorn, D. K. and Gross, S.,** Vitamin E dependent anaemia in the premature infant. II. Interrelationships between gestational age and absorption of vitamin E, *J. Pediatr.,* 79, 581, 1971.

76. **Oski, F. A. and Barness, L. A.,** Vitamin E deficiency: a previously unrecognized cause of hemolytic anemia in the premature infant, *J. Pediatr.,* 70, 211, 1967.

77. **Williams, M. L., Shott, R. J., O'Neal, P. L., and Oski, F. A.,** Role of dietary iron and fat on vitamin E deficiency anemia of infancy, *N. Engl. J. Med.,* 292, 887, 1975.

78. **Fermanian, J., Salmon, D., Olive, G., Zambrowski, S., Rossier, A., and Caldera, R.,** Vitamin E versus placebo: a double-blind comparative trial in the low birth weight infant in the seventh week of life, *Nouv. Rev. Fr. Hematol.,* 16, 246, 1976.

79. **Jansson, L., Holmberg, L., Nilsson, B., and Johansson, B.,** Vitamin E requirements of preterm infants, *Acta Paediatr. Scand.,* 67, 459, 1978.

80. **Panos, T. C., Stinnett, B., Zapata, G., Eminians, J., Marasigan, B. V., and Beard, A. G.,** Vitamin E and linoleic acid in the feeding of premature infants, *Am. J. Clin. Nutr.,* 21, 15, 1968.

81. **Gross, S. J., Landaw, S. A., and Oski, F. A.,** Vitamin E and neonatal hemolysis, *Pediatrics,* 59, 995, 1977.

82. **Blanchette, V., Bell, E., Nahmias, C., Garnett, S., Milner, R., and Zipursky, A.,** A randomized control trial of vitamin E therapy in the prevention of anemia in low birth weight infants, *Pediatr. Res.,* 14, 591, 1980.

83. **Bell, E. F. and Filer, L. J., Jr.,** The role of vitamin E in the nutrition of premature infants, *Am. J. Clin. Nutr.,* 34, 414, 1981.

84. **Zipursky, A.,** Vitamin E deficiency anemia in newborn infants, *Clin. Perinatol.,* 11, 393, 1984.

85. **Smith, K. A. and Mengel, C. E.,** Association of iron-dextran-induced hemolysis and lipid peroxidation in mice, *J. Lab. Clin. Med.,* 72, 505, 1968.

86. **Tollerz, G. and Lannek, N.,** Protection against iron toxicity in vitamin E-deficient piglets and mice by vitamin E and synthetic antioxidants, *Nature,* 201, 846, 1964.

87. **Varga, S. J., Matkovics, B., Pataki, L., Monar, A., and Novak, Z.,** Comparison of antioxidant red blood cell enzymes in premature and full-term neonates, *Clin. Chim. Acta,* 147, 191, 1985.

88. **Hassan, H., Hashim, S. A., Van Itallie, T. B., and Sebrell, W. H.,** Syndrome in premature infants associated with low plasma vitamin E levels and high polyunsaturated fatty acid diet, *Am. J. Clin. Nutr.,* 19, 147, 1966.

89. American Academy of Pediatrics Committee on Nutrition, Nutritional needs of low-birth-weight infants, *Pediatrics,* 75, 976, 1985.

90. **Jansson, L., Homberg, L., and Åkesson, B.,** Vitamin E and fatty acid composition in human milk, *Am. J. Clin. Nutr.,* 34, 8, 1981.

91. **Gross, S. J. and Gabriel, E.,** Vitamin E status in preterm infants fed human milk or infant formula, *J. Pediatr.,* 106, 635, 1985.

Chapter 5

IRON IN HUMAN MILK AND COW'S MILK — EFFECTS OF BINDING LIGANDS ON BIOAVAILABILITY

Bo Lönnerdal

TABLE OF CONTENTS

I. INTRODUCTION

A low incidence of anemia in breast-fed infants at least up to 6 months and possibly even up to 9 months of age, combined with a low concentration of iron in human milk as compared to most infant formulas, early led to the suggestion of high bioavailability of iron from human milk. Studies in infants using radioisotope measurements as well as the conventional balance method, seemed to corroborate this suggestion; however, iron absorption in infants is highly variable depending on iron status, other dietary components, etc. and the number of subjects studied to date is very low, making evaluations difficult. It is possible that when the techniques of using and analyzing stable isotopes becomes more available to researchers, further studies on iron absorption and metabolism in infants can be done.

At this time, there seems to be a general consensus that although there are only a limited number of studies on iron absorption in infants, the data support a high bioavailability of iron from human milk; however, there is very little information on the mechanism(s) behind this high iron absorption.

The purpose of this chapter is to describe the various ligands binding in human milk and how they compare to ligands in cow's milk, and in light of this, discuss the possible mechanisms assuring a high uptake of iron from human milk by the infant. Factors affecting human milk iron concentration as well as other milk sources used in infant feeding are also discussed.

II. FORMS OF IRON IN HUMAN MILK

A. PROTEIN-BOUND IRON

In biological tissues and fluids, iron is almost exclusively bound to proteins, such as hemoglobin, myoglobin, transferrin, and ferritin. Low molecular weight complexes of iron are present in very low concentrations, but are believed to serve as important intermediary forms of iron being transferred from one protein to another. The proteins binding iron have developed an affinity toward either ferrous ($+$II) or ferric iron ($+$III) and it is likely that the low molecular weight complexes make iron available for redox reactions necessary for the transfer of iron between proteins.

In human milk, it was early found that a large fraction of iron is bound to proteins,[1] and subsequently that lactoferrin (lactotransferrin) is the major iron-binding protein.[2,3] When human milk was separated by ultracentrifugation and ultrafiltration, approximately 30% of the total iron content was found to be bound to lactoferrin.[3-5] Lactoferrin is a glycoprotein with a molecular weight of 82,400.[6] It consists of 703 amino acids and two glycan moieties linked to asparagine residues. Similar to transferrin, lactoferrin can bind two ferric ions concomitant with two carbonate or bicarbonate ions and the molecule appears to be the result of a gene duplication resulting in two structurally similar half-molecules.[7] The two carbohydrate side chains of human lactoferrin consist of N-acetyllactosamine-type glycans with fucose, galactose, and sialic acid as terminals (Figure 1). These glycans are different than the glycans found in transferrin, that have only sialic acid as terminal monosaccharides. Another difference between lactoferrin and transferrin is the considerably stronger dissociation constant for the iron-lactoferrin complex, 10^{30}, as compared to iron-transferrin, 10^{27}.[2] This difference in affinity toward iron results in a difference in pH-dependent iron release. While transferrin-iron will become released at pH 5, a considerably lower pH ($<$3) is necessary to release iron from lactoferrin.[2] The strong dissociation constant for lactoferrin-iron can be used in support of the physiological functions proposed for lactoferrin (see below). In the light of the strong affinity of lactoferrin to iron, the observation of a very low degree of saturation of lactoferrin with iron may appear inconsistent. It should be recognized, however, that lactoferrin is present in human milk at a concentration of 10 to

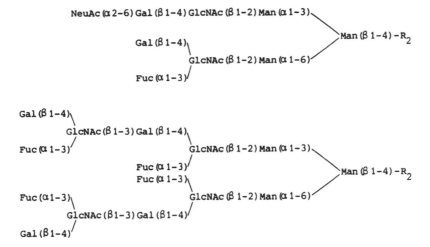

FIGURE 1. Primary structure of human lactoferrin glycans.[9] (From Goavec, M., and Montreil, J., *Proteins of Iron Storage and Transport*, Spik, G., Montreil, J., Crichton, R. R., and Mazurier, J., Eds., Elsevier, Amsterdam, 1985, 47. With permission.)

30 μM while iron is present in a concentration of 2 to 6 μM. Thus, even if *all* iron in human milk would be bound to lactoferrin, it would only be saturated to about 20%.[3] Since iron in human milk is also bound to other ligands to at least 60 to 70%, it is obvious that at most only 6 to 8% of the iron-binding capacity of lactoferrin in human milk is utilized. A remaining question, however, is why only 30 to 40% of iron in human milk is bound to lactoferrin with its tenacity for iron? There may be two reasons for this finding. First, low molecular weight ligands capable of coordinating iron are present in concentrations considerably higher than that of lactoferrin. For example, citrate, a chelator of iron, is present in human milk at a concentration of about 3000 μM.[10] Consequently, the equilibrium of the binding between iron and citrate and iron and lactoferrin is pushed toward the former complex. Secondly, iron in the lipid compartment (see below) may be inaccessible for ligand exchange due to the hydrophobic nature of the lipid fraction. Thus, the facilitory role of low molecular weight ligands in iron transfer reactions among iron-binding proteins may be abolished by hydrophobic barriers.

The concentration of lactoferrin is high in colostrum and subsequently decreases (see below). There is still some controversy with regard to the effect of maternal nutrition on the concentration of lactoferrin in humans. While Prentice et al.[11] found similar levels of lactoferrin in milk from Gambian women of poor nutritional status as compared to other women, Houghton et al.[12] found lower lactoferrin levels in milk from women who had low (<90%) weight for height than in control women. On the other hand, Fransson et al.[13] found higher levels of lactoferrin in anemic lactating women in India than in nonanemic controls. Thus, further studies are needed on the regulation of lactoferrin synthesis in the mammary gland.

Another human milk protein that contains iron as an integral part is xanthine oxidase (EC 1.2.3.2). This enzyme consists of two identical polypeptide chains with a molecular weight of 149,000 and contains a flavin cofactor with eight atoms of iron and two atoms of molybdenum.[14] Xanthine oxidase is membrane-bound and appears to be primarily bound to the outer fat globule membrane of the lipid droplets in human milk.[15] Up to 30% of the total iron content of human milk is found in the lipid fraction and solubilization/chromatography studies indicate that most of this iron is bound to xanthine oxidase. Since the concentration of fat in human milk varies within a feed, milk iron concentration also varies.[16,17] In fore-milk iron concentration is low, while it is high in hind-milk (Figure 2). The

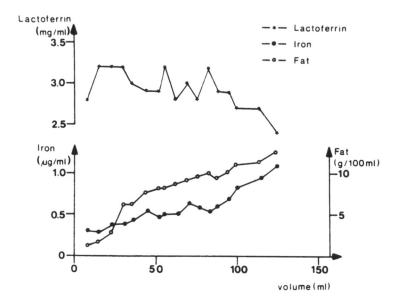

FIGURE 2.   Concentration of iron, fat, and lactoferrin in human milk during the course of a single nursing.[2]

biological function of xanthine oxidase in milk has not yet been elucidated, although it is known that the enzyme has NADH-cytochrome *c* reductase activity.[18] The biochemistry of xanthine oxidase is very complex; the enzyme also exists in a dehydrogenase form, in several isoenzymes, and in "de-sulfo" and "de-molybdo" forms.[14] The milk lipid xanthine oxidase is present in the oxidase form and is structurally and functionally similar to the xanthine oxidase of the endothelial cells of capillaries.[18] Although xanthine oxidase can promote lipid peroxidation when incubated with hypoxanthine *in vitro,* this does not appear to occur *in vivo.*[18]

Ferritin is also present in human milk, at a concentration of 20 to 30 µg/l.[19,20] While ferritin fully saturated with iron might contribute significantly to milk iron, serum ferritin is only saturated to a low degree and it is unlikely that ferritin in milk has any nutritional significance.

B. IRON COMPLEXED TO LOW MOLECULAR WEIGHT COMPOUNDS

Part of the iron in human milk can be separated by ultrafiltration.[3,4] Using an ultrafiltration membrane with a molecular weight cut-off of 10,000, about 30% of the iron passed through the membrane. The compounds to which iron in this fraction is complexed have not yet been identified with any certainty, although our preliminary data strongly indicate that a major part is complexed to citrate (unpublished observations). We have previously identified citrate as the major low molecular weight ligand binding zinc in human milk.[21] Iron coelutes with zinc and citrate when human milk ultrafiltrates are chromatographed on Sephadex G-15. Furthermore, when citrate is degraded by citrate lyase and malate dehydrogenase, the elution position of zinc and iron is changed (unpublished observations). These observations are in agreement with the findings of Morley and Bezkorovainy,[22] who suggested that the low molecular weight iron complex in hepatocytes is ferric citrate. Recently, Mulligan et al.[23] fractionated low molecular weight iron complexes from several rat tissues. One of the iron complexes found had a molecular weight of 350, which is consistent with a ferric citrate complex. Thus, it is possible that ferric citrate is a pool of non-heme iron which is present in several tissues and fluids. Although the size of this pool in general may be small, it can be hypothesized to function as a "shuttle-bus" for iron in cellular iron transport. In human

TABLE 1
Concentration and Distribution of Iron in Milk of Various Species

Species	Fe Colostrum μg/ml	Mature milk μg/ml	Casein %	Whey %	Fat %
Human	0.8	0.2—0.4	2—14	65—81	19—26
Cow	0.2	0.1—0.2	61—73	9—15	13—18
Goat	1.4	0.3—0.5	33—49	28—51	12—20
Sheep	0.5	0.2—0.5	37—49	25—36	20—32
Horse	1.3	0.3—1.0	30—80	5—33	10—43
Pig	1.3	1—2	32—52	35—50	18—43
Rat	6.6	5—10	34—42	17—65	3—25
Dog	10.7	2—8	63—79	6—26	5—19
Cat	4.1	1—4	4—68	40—85	2—18

Adapted from Lönnerdal, B., Keen, C. L., and Hurley, L. S., *Trace Element Metabolism in Man and Animals (TEMA)-4*, Howell, J. McC., Gawthorne, J. M., and White, C. L., Eds., Griffen Press, Netly, South Australia, 1981, 249.

milk, however, the finding of a relatively large fraction of iron in this pool may be a consequence of the high concentration of citrate produced by the Golgi.

III. IRON CONTENT OF HUMAN MILK

A. VARIATION DURING LACTATION

The concentration of iron in milk produced by well-nourished women of fairly homogeneous socioeconomic status has been shown to vary during lactation. Siimes et al.[24] showed in a study of Finnish women that milk iron was around 0.5 to 0.6 mg/l in early lactation (0 to 2 weeks), 0.4 to 0.5 mg/l up to 3 months of lactation, and 0.2 to 0.4 mg/l thereafter. There was a continuous decrease in milk iron with the most dramatic decrease in early lactation. Similar results with regard to both concentration and developmental patterns have been obtained for milk from other groups of women.[25-28] While most studies show similar concentrations of iron in milk produced during early lactation (Table 1), two studies report considerably higher iron concentrations.[29,30] It is not yet known whether the contrasting results were due to methodological problems or to different populations. It is hoped that the milk trace element standard recently introduced by the National Bureau of Standards will help to elucidate these discrepancies.

The reasons for the longitudinal changes in milk iron concentration during lactation are not known. It is interesting to note, however, that the pattern for milk iron concentration during lactation is very similar to that for lactoferrin concentration (Figure 3). It is possible that lactoferrin, synthesized by the mammary gland, is acting as a sequestering agent for iron entering the mammary epithelial cells. The amount of iron in xanthine oxidase may be regulated by lipid synthesis or not regulated at all but a constant function of plasma membranes surrounding lipid droplets. Iron complexed to low molecular weight complexes, in turn, may be a function of the amount of iron initially sequestered by lactoferrin or a function of citrate concentration/Golgi activity. Thus, considerably more information regarding iron transport into milk and metabolic activity of the mammary gland is needed before the factors determining the variation in milk iron during lactation can be elucidated.

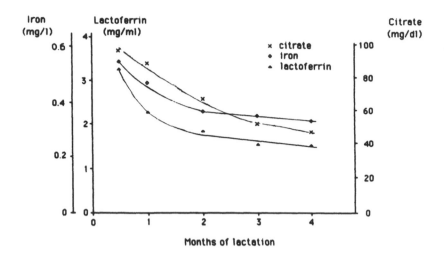

FIGURE 3.   Iron, lactoferrin, and citrate concentration of human milk during the course of lactation. (Adapted from References 24, 31, and 32.)

B. EFFECT OF MATERNAL IRON STATUS ON MILK IRON CONCENTRATION

The incidence of iron deficiency anemia is high in infants in developing countries,[33] while infants in developed countries rarely become anemic.[34] There are several reasons for these differences (as described in other chapters), but a case could potentially be made for differences in milk iron concentrations being part of the causative factor. Women in developing countries are often anemic both during pregnancy and lactation, while women in industrialized countries frequently use iron supplements during both these periods. Thus, if milk iron concentration were reflective of maternal iron status, the iron nutrition of the nursing infant could be affected; however, most studies to date suggest that maternal iron status does not affect milk iron concentration. It should be cautioned, however, that the number and extent of studies carried out to date has been very limited and that it is difficult to make any firm conclusions.[10]

The most common approach that has been used in studies on milk iron concentration is that of correlating iron intake to milk iron concentration. However, this approach has several drawbacks: (1) if the iron status of the mother is adequate, homeostatic regulation of iron absorption limits the amount of iron taken up by the intestine and subsequently being circulated — thus, the amount of iron available for transport into the mammary gland is not reflective of maternal intake; (2) if the mother is iron deficient, iron absorption is increased as a compensatory mechanism — thus, the amount of iron available for the mammary gland may be higher than indicated by maternal intake. In addition, we do not know the relative priorities of iron-demanding activities in various tissues of the body. Bearing these cautions in mind, it is not surprising that most studies fail to correlate milk iron to maternal iron intake.

In a study by Picciano and Guthrie,[35] no effect of iron intake on milk iron concentration was found. However, these women had iron intakes of at least 30 mg/d and 74% of them were taking iron supplements. Milk iron levels in this study were low, which was explained by the use of fore-milk samples. Analytical problems may also explain the very high levels of iron reported by Karmarkar and Ramakrishnan.[36] These authors did not find a correlation between maternal iron intake and iron in milk from women who had nursed for 1 to 31 months. These women had a high intake of iron (39 to 65 mg/d) and no correlation between dietary iron and milk iron was found. Vuori et al.[37] did not find any correlation between iron intake and milk iron concentration in Finnish women, however, 60% of these women were taking iron supplements. Similarly, Finley et al.[28] did not find any correlation between dietary iron and milk in a group of women having iron intakes at least 200% of the RDA for iron.

Very high levels of iron intake do not appear to affect milk iron concentration. Fransson et al.[38] compared a group of Ethiopian women with iron intakes higher than 200 mg/d with a group of Swedish women. Milk iron concentrations were similar in the two groups. Iron status was not assessed, but it can be assumed that it was good to excellent in both groups. It should be noted that the high iron intake of the Ethiopian women was due to high intake of the staple cereal teff, which becomes contaminated by iron-rich soil. It has been shown that the bioavailability of such iron is very low[39] and consequently the amount of iron absorbed may have been substantially lower than indicated by the dietary level.

The potential effects of maternal iron deficiency on milk iron concentration have been studied in a few limited investigations. Murray et al.[29] analyzed iron in milk samples from Nigerian women that did not receive iron supplements or meat (the proportion of meat in the diet consumed is important to consider since heme iron is considerably better absorbed than non-heme iron). At both 2 weeks and 6 months postpartum, women that were either anemic (Hgb $\leq$ 10 g/dl), normal (Hgb 10 to 12 g/dl), or "over-loaded" (Hgb $\geq$ 12 g/dl), produced milk with similar iron concentrations. The different hemoglobin values were also reflected in widely different transferrin saturation (6, 27, and 64%, respectively). The values obtained for milk iron concentration in early lactation, about 1.2 mg/l, were considerably higher than in most other studies and methodological problems cannot be ruled out; however, even if the milk iron levels were overestimated, it appears that low levels of circulating iron do not reduce milk iron levels.

A recent study of Indian anemic women implies a positive effect of iron deficiency on milk iron concentration.[13] Women with hemoglobin concentrations <8.0 g/dl had milk iron concentrations significantly higher than women having hemoglobin values >11.0 g/dl. In addition, the concentration of lactoferrin was significantly higher in milk from anemic women as compared to nonanemic women. It should be noted that the hematological parameters were assessed at delivery and milk samples were taken at $\leq$ 2 weeks postpartum. It was not stated in the paper, but from an ethical point of view, it is likely that women that were found to be severely anemic at delivery immediately were supplemented with iron. Although no effect on hemoglobin values are expected in 2 weeks or less, increases would be expected in circulating levels of iron and consequently transferrin saturation. As stated earlier, the mechanisms of iron transfer from serum into milk are largely unknown; however, transferrin receptors have been found on the plasma membrane of cells from lactating rabbits[40] and rats.[41] Therefore, a sudden increase in transferrin receptor-mediated iron uptake may have led to a high transfer of iron into milk. The possibility that the higher levels of lactoferrin are responsible for a higher transfer of iron into milk, regardless of circulating iron levels, also needs to be considered.

In a study of iron concentration in milk from lactating Swiss women, Celada et al.[42] found no correlation between hemoglobin levels, serum ferritin, or transferrin saturation with milk iron; however, mean hemoglobin concentration was 13.1 g/dl and the range was 11 to 15 g/dl. Consequently, this group of women was relatively homogeneous and the women overall had good iron status. It should also be recognized that these women had been taking 100 mg of iron per day during pregnancy and milk samples were taken 10 d postpartum. Therefore, the data provided may be of limited value when assessing the correlation between maternal hematological parameters and milk iron.

It is evident that there are limitations with regard to the extent of dietary iron deficiency and excess that can be studied in humans. There are ethical considerations when studying severely anemic women and the time period for which these women can be left unsupplemented. When evaluating efficacy of various iron supplements, potential interactive effects on other nutrients as well as other safety aspects need to be considered. Consequently, some of the crucial questions concerning milk iron regulation have to be addressed in experimental animals.

In the rat, it has been shown that iron supplementation can increase milk iron concentration. Ezekiel and Morgan[43] gave rats ferrous ammonium sulfate as a supplement in the drinking water. Iron concentration of milk from rats receiving a high iron intake (0.3 g of iron per liter) was about 8 mg/l while milk from control rats had an iron concentration of about 4.5 mg/l. However, tissue iron concentrations were similar in pups from iron-supplemented and control dams. Keen et al.[44] supplemented lactating rats with iron (0.9 g/l) as ferrous nitrilotriacetic acid (NTA) and found significantly higher iron concentration (7 mg/l) in milk from supplemented dams as compared to control dams (4 mg/l). The chelating agent NTA is known to readily donate iron to transferrin and consequently it is likely that circulating iron levels and transferrin saturation were high in supplemented rats. Liver iron concentrations of supplemented lactating dams as well as their suckling pups were significantly higher than those of control dams and pups. Anaokar and Garry[45] studied the effects of feeding a high level of iron in the diet (2500 μg/g diet) to lactating rats. Liver and plasma ferritin values were higher and TIBC lower in supplemented dams as compared to control rats. Iron concentration was higher (about 12 mg/l) in milk from iron-supplemented dams than from control rats (8 mg/l). Thus, it appears that iron concentration of rat milk can be increased by high levels of iron in the diet or the drinking water.

Iron deficiency in lactating rats, as induced by repeated bleeding, has been shown to result in decreased milk iron concentration.[43] Rats that had been bled (Hgb = 11 g/dl), had at 16 d of lactation a milk iron concentration of about 3 mg/l while in control rats (Hgb = 13 g/dl) milk iron level was about 4.5 mg/l. It should be cautioned, however, that the large number of mammary glands and the very high rate of milk production in the rat, makes milk assimilation a much more demanding process than in the human. Sherman et al.[46] fed rats a diet deficient in iron (5 μ/g diet) from conception to day 18 of lactation. Milk iron concentration was 3.1 mg/l in deficient dams and 9.4 mg/l in control dams (receiving 300 μg iron per gram diet). Anaokar and Garry[45] also fed rats an iron-deficient diet, but this diet was introduced at day 3 of lactation. The iron level of the deficient diet was not given, but liver and plasma ferritin and hemoglobin levels were lower in iron-deficient dams as compared to rats fed the control diet (250 μg iron per gram diet). At day 19 of lactation, iron concentration in milk from iron-deficient dams was lower (about 3.5 mg/l) than in milk from control rats (about 8.0 mg/l). Thus, in both studies in which iron-deficient diets were used, milk iron levels were reduced to about 50% of control levels, even if the deficient diet was not introduced until day 3 of lactation.

C. IRON IN MILK OF OTHER SPECIES

Cow's milk is commonly used as a protein source for infant formulas, although it is recommended that cow's milk as such should not be used during the first 6 months of life. Hence, the amount of iron provided by cow's milk as well as the ligands inhibiting to promoting iron absorption are relevant for our discussion on human milk. Another reason for discussing iron and its localization in milk from other species is the need for developing animal models proper to use in both evaluating formulas as well as in basic research on the molecular mechanisms underlying iron absorption in infants.

Iron in cow's milk is primarily bound to the casein fraction (61 to 73%) and relatively little iron (9 to 15%) is found in the whey fraction (Table 1). Similar to human milk, a significant portion of the iron is found in the fat fraction, 13 to 18%, most likely bound to xanthine oxidase.[48] The localization of iron within the casein fraction has been studied by Hegenauer et al.[49] These investigators found that iron was associated with negatively charged phosphoserine groups located on the β-casein subunits of bovine casein. Within the whey fraction, it is likely that lactoferrin is binding some of the iron; although the lactoferrin concentration of cow's milk is considerably lower than that of human milk, the 0.01 to 0.1 mg/ml present in cow's milk potentially could bind 0.01 to 0.14 μg iron per milliliter of milk. Since the total concentration of iron in cow's milk is 0.1 to 0.2 μg/ml, a substantial proportion of iron in the whey could be bound to lactoferrin. It has been shown, however, that about half of the whey iron in cow's milk is associated to low molecular weight ligands.[4] Therefore, besides a larger proportion of iron within the casein fraction, the distribution of iron in cow's milk is not fundamentally different than that of human milk.

Milk from species other than the human and the cow is generally higher in iron concentration (Table 1). In all species, however, iron concentration of colostrum is higher than in mature milk. As the protein concentration of colostrum also is higher than in mature milk, it is logical that iron that is primarily bound to proteins in milk would be higher in concentration in colostrum. Although this correlation cannot be made in general when comparing species — cow's milk has three times the protein concentration of human milk but lower iron concentration — it is evident that our knowledge regarding the factors controlling milk iron concentration is limited.

Since milk from virtually all mammalian species contains a higher concentration casein than human milk,[54] it is likely that casein will be a major iron-binding protein in milk from most species. As seen in Table 1, this has been shown for most species studied. The major iron-binding protein of whey, however, varies among species. Human, cow, sow, and guinea pig milk all have lactoferrin as the primary iron-binding protein in their whey, while other species, such as rodents have transferrin as the major whey iron-binding protein.[55] Transferrin in milk is immunologically similar to transferrin in serum and it has been thought that transferrin in milk originates from serum. Jordan and Morgan[56] showed, however, that while some serum proteins, such as serum albumin and IgG are transferred into milk to a limited extent, transferrin is synthesized by the mammary gland to a substantial degree. Recently, Leclercq et al.[57] showed that the glycans of serum transferrin and milk transferrin are different, supporting local synthesis of transferrin in the mammary gland. Interestingly, it was found that mouse milk contains both lactoferrin and transferrin in high concentrations. The reason why some species synthesize lactoferrin in the mammary cell and others transferrin is not known.

When choosing an animal model to study iron in milk and its bioavailability, it is apparent that the rat with its high milk iron concentration, comparatively high proportion of iron in casein and low in the fat fraction, as well as having transferrin as the major milk iron-binding protein is not ideal. The pig, although having somewhat higher iron concentration, appears a better choice since lactoferrin is the dominant whey iron-binding protein.[58] On the other hand, the piglet has a very high requirement for iron during the neonatal period. Another species that appears similar to the human with regard to iron in milk and iron metabolism is the Rhesus monkey.[59] The concentration of lactoferrin in Rhesus milk is similar to that of human milk and the protein cross-reacts with the human lactoferrin antibody. In addition, like human lactoferrin, Rhesus lactoferrin has fucose-containing glycan moieties, while bovine lactoferrin glycans do not contain fucose (Figure 1). This latter property has been shown to be crucial for the binding of lactoferrin to mucosal receptors (see below). The monkey has also been demonstrated to absorb ferrous and ferric iron at a similar ratio as that found for humans.[60] Therefore, it is likely that the Rhesus monkey can serve as a useful model for studies in iron absorption from milk.

IV. BIOAVAILABILITY OF IRON FROM HUMAN MILK

A. IRON STATUS OF BREAST-FED INFANTS

Although it has long been known that the incidence of anemia is low for breast-fed infants and considerably higher for infants fed cow's milk or cow's milk formula, only a

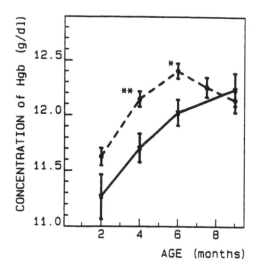

FIGURE 4. Changes in hemoglobin concentrations of exclusively breast-fed infants (dashed line) and infants fed iron-supplemented formula (solid line).[66]

limited number of studies have directly addressed the question of how long breast milk *only* can cover the iron needs of infants. In 1928, MacKay[61] studied infants exclusively breast-fed up to the age of 7 months and compared these infants with a group of artificially fed infants. The breast-fed infants consistently had higher hemoglobin levels than the artificially fed group, although this difference decreased after other foods were introduced. In a limited study of four infants, McMillan et al.[62] found that these infants that had been exclusively breast-fed for 8 to 18 months (!) had normal hemoglobin and serum iron levels. Using more strict criteria to also assess iron deficiency without anemia (MCV, transferrin saturation, serum ferritin), Saarinen[63] followed 56 exclusively breast-fed infants and found no indication of iron deficiency at 6 months. At 9 months of age, however, about 4% of the breast-fed group showed signs of iron deficiency. It is not known if this higher incidence of iron deficiency at 9 months of age is a function of the low iron concentration of human milk at this stage of lactation, the introduction of solid foods reducing the high bioavailability of human milk iron,[64] or a combination of both. Picciano and Deering[65] followed iron status of infants receiving various feeding regimens during the first year of life. Infants that were exclusively breast-fed for 3 months had excellent iron status at 6 and 9 months, although it should be emphasized that these infants were receiving substantial quantities of iron from iron-fortified cereals from 3 months of age.

Exclusive breast feeding for prolonged periods of time may not be common in the U.S., but it should be recognized that this occurs in some segments of the U.S. population, and is relatively common in Europe and in developing countries. It is, therefore, important to establish the adequacy of breast milk to provide iron to the infant. Siimes et al.[66] studied 36 infants that were exclusively breast-fed for 9 months. At 4 and 6 months of age, iron status of breast-fed infants was higher than that of infants fed iron-supplemented formula and solid food (Figure 4). At 9 months of age, however, the breast-fed infants tended to have lower values of MCV, serum ferritin, transferrin saturation, and serum iron. Hemoglobin values, however, were similar to those of controls, i.e., infants weaned prior to $3^{1}/_{2}$ months of age and receiving iron-supplemented formulas and foods. Thus, it appears that up to 6 months of age, breast-fed infants receive sufficient amounts of iron, but after that supplementation with iron is advisable. A recent study by Duncan et al.[67] corroborates these conclusions; 33 infants exclusively breast-fed for 6 months showed no sign of anemia

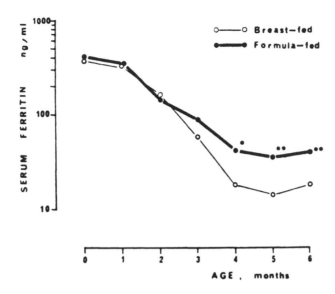

FIGURE 5. Changes in serum ferritin concentration in breast-fed infants and infants fed iron-supplemented formula.[68]

and only a low frequency (7%) of low serum ferritin levels. Low-birth-weight infants, however, may have a higher requirement for iron because of lower stores of iron caused by prematurity and because of rapid growth rate. Iwai et al.[68] showed that such infants have lower iron status at 4 months of age than infants fed iron-supplemented formula (Figure 5).

It should be recognized that the infants in the studies discussed were all healthy and had normal growth patterns. Our knowledge of iron needs of infants with compromised health is much more limited. Reeves et al.[69] showed that repeated minor infections caused a higher incidence of iron deficiency in infants, indicating a higher iron requirement during illness. Another situation to consider is that during rapid growth, especially during refeeding from malnutrition, trace element needs are higher because of the large amounts of new tissue laid down. Therefore, growth spurts may put higher demands on dietary iron. Several other cases can be made illustrating the fact that breast-feeding for 6 months should not be taken as a guarantee for avoiding iron deficiency, although the majority of normal, healthy infants will receive adequate iron nutrition from human milk up to 6 months of age.

These observations on hematological indices of breast-fed infants argue against the recommendations on iron supplementation by Fomon and Strauss[70] which were based on calculations of the use of iron stores, need for iron for anabolic needs, and available iron provided by human milk. It seems evident that some of the parameters used in these calculations must be wrong and further studies on their validity are needed. Other investigators have also attempted to theoretically calculate the adequacy of milk iron for the breast-fed infant.[71,72] These authors arrived at different conclusions, fueling a discussion.[73]

It appears evident that further studies on the bioavailability of iron from human milk and formula are necessary to answer some of these questions.

B. ABSORPTION STUDIES IN INFANTS

The number of studies directly measuring iron absorption in infants is very limited. Balance studies have been used to obtain some assessment of iron requirements of infants, but this technique does not measure absorption as the endogenous losses cannot be determined. In addition, the balance periods used are usually too short for estimation of absorbed iron. Excluding the balance method as a tool in measuring iron absorption, the investigator is left with the choice of isotope labeling and indirect determination by mathematical modeling. The use of animal models can give complementary information with regard to mechanisms of absorption. These options will be described below.

One of the first studies of iron absorption from milk in infants using a radioactive isotope of iron, ^{59}Fe, was performed in 1958 by Schulz and Smith.[74] In this study, absorption of the radiolabel from cow's milk was determined in infants and children 3 months to 15 years of age by measuring fecal radioiron excretion and hemoglobin ^{59}Fe incorporation. Both methods used appeared to yield similar results and are in fact both still being used. Although not specified, it appears that only four of the subjects were infants (<12 months of age). Iron absorption was found to be age-dependent with five children having a mean iron absorption of 9.1% from milk and adult men a mean absorption of 2.8%. Schulz and Smith were aware of the dilemma of using an extrinsic label added to milk to assess bioavailability of all iron in milk and, therefore, also used intrinsically labeled cow's milk, i.e., lactating cows were injected intravenously with ^{59}Fe and labeled milk was collected and homogenized. Results were similar for milk labeled by both methods; 10.6% absorbed from extrinsically labeled milk and 9.1% from intrinsically labeled milk. Unfortunately, these were two different groups of infants and although their age range was similar, it is not known if their iron status was. The results of the study indicate that iron-deficient children absorbed more iron than children with normal hemoglobin values. It is known that iron status may have a more pronounced effect on iron absorption than dietary composition.[75] A major conclusion of their study (which still is valid) was that iron absorption from cow's milk is low and that "many infants would have to absorb more iron than is present in cow's milk to avoid not only iron deficiency but also frank iron-deficiency anemia."

Garby and Sjölin[76] also used radiolabeled (^{59}Fe) milk to study iron absorption in infants by the fecal excretion method. The subjects in their study were younger (10 to 90 d) than those in the study of Schulz and Smith and a larger number of infants (n = 12) was used. The absorption values for these infants were substantially higher than in the older infants in the previous study, further emphasizing the effect of age on iron absorption. These investigators also found that iron absorption was negatively correlated to the amount of iron in the test meal given. A drawback of this study is that three different diets were used — human milk, cow's milk, and infant formula — all with different iron concentration. Since it was not specified which infant received each type of diet, it is impossible to assess the effect of diet vs. iron concentration. The large variability in iron absorption values in this age group was a noticeable finding.

The effect of volume of milk ingested with the test diet was assessed by Heinrich et al.[77] They found that iron absorption in infants, as measured by the extrinsic tag method, was 18.3% from 5 mg of ferrous iron in a test dose alone and 3.8% from the same test dose given with 50 ml of cow's milk. This comparison is not feasible, though, as not only the larger volume but also the cow's milk could have affected iron absorption. Garby and Sjölin,[76] however, found higher iron absorption values when the test meal was given in between meals as compared to with a meal. Consistent with previous reports, Heinrich et al.[77] also found that iron absorption from a 10-mg Fe^{2+} dose was 7.6% as compared to 18% from a 5-mg dose.

The first study to directly assess absorption of radioiron from human milk in infants was performed by Saarinen et al.[78] The infants were 6 to 7 months old and had been either exclusively breast-fed or weaned early to a home-prepared cow's milk formula. The test dose of ^{59}Fe in water was given either during a breast feeding or after 3 h of fasting and absorption was measured in a whole body counter. Mean iron absorption from human milk was 49%, from the test dose in fasted breast-fed infants 38%, and from the test dose in fasted formula-fed infants 19% (Figure 6). Although the variation in absorption values was large, the values were significantly different from each other. Their conclusions were that iron absorption from human milk is high and that there is some "preconditioning" effect

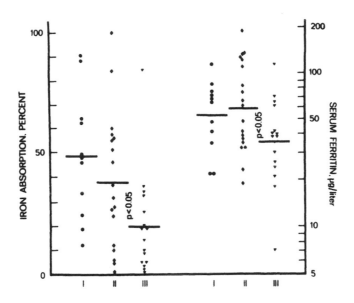

FIGURE 6. Iron absorption (left) and serum ferritin values (right) in infants. Group I: Breast milk diet, iron given with breast feeding. Group II: Breast milk diet, iron given after a fast. Group III: Cow milk diet, iron given after a fast.[78]

of breast feeding that facilitates iron absorption in these infants even in a fasted stage. The "true" absorption value in the formula-fed infants may be lower as these infants were shown to have lower ferritin levels than the breast-fed infants and, therefore, could be expected to have increased iron absorption due to homeostatic regulation. It should be emphasized that these infants were fasted for 3 h; although it is implicated in their discussion, it cannot be ascertained that the upper gastrointestinal tract was "cleaned" from the previous meal at this time point. We have recently shown in a 7-month-old infant that duodenal aspirates taken 3 h post feeding contain substantial quantities of the previous meal.[79] Thus, it is possible that breast milk and formula, respectively, were labeled by the test dose given 3 h later. This might explain why there was no significant difference in iron absorption for the fed breast-fed group vs. the "fasted" breast-fed group. The value for iron absorption in the fasted formula-fed group is also similar to that obtained for infant formula which is not fortified with iron.[80]

Because of concern for exposing infants to radioisotopes, the number of studies using such isotopes will be very limited. One approach to avoid this problem is to use a stable isotope of iron. Janghorbani et al.[80] have used ^{58}Fe to study the absorption of iron in 4-month-old infants that were fasted for 2 h. Although this was a limited feasibility study in four infants only, the absorption values calculated from hemoglobin ^{58}Fe incorporation data, 6.5 to 14.7%, were in agreement with those obtained by using radioisotopes in infants fed infant formula.[81] The authors point out that their results are based on the assumption that all absorbed iron is incorporated into hemoglobin, which has not yet been proven for infants. A more reliable method would be based on fecal collections, but this may require hospitalization of the infants. Also, iron absorption needs to be relatively high (>10%) to assure adequate labeling of the hemoglobin; the amount of label must be kept low in order to not substantially alter the iron concentration of the food item to be tested. Taking the above considerations into account, however, it appears likely that this may become a valuable and safe technique of studying iron absorption in infants. Recently, Fairweather-Tait et al.[82] also used ^{58}Fe to study iron absorption in infants. They found a high absorption of iron from formula, approximately 45%, with a high degree of individual variation.

Another approach to assessing iron bioavailability from infant foods is to use human adults. Techniques for studying iron absorption in adults by using radioisotopes have been well developed and are frequently used. These techniques use hemoglobin incorporation or whole body counting or a combination of both using two radioisotopes of iron.[83] This approach was used by McMillan et al.[62] who gave fasted human adults human milk or cow's milk extrinsically labeled with ^{59}Fe. Incorporation of iron into red blood cells was found to be 20.8% from human milk and 13.6% from cow's milk. Making the two assumptions that RBC incorporation is about 80% of absorbed iron in the adult and that iron absorption of infants is about twice that of adults, iron absorption in infants from human milk and cow's milk would be 50% and 34%, respectively. It could be argued that the value for iron absorption from cow's milk may have been overestimated. The adult with fully developed gastrointestinal function can be expected to completely digest cow's milk casein while this may not be true in infants.[84] If there is a negative effect of casein on iron absorption, it is likely to be more pronounced in infants than in adults (see below).

A remaining question is whether the extrinsic label of iron used in the above studies is equilibrating with the native iron in milk diets. This is a necessary prerequisite for the methods used and remains to be proven. We have previously shown that although isotope equilibrium appears to be achieved for the label and cold iron in cow's milk, it does not appear to occur for human milk.[85] Rather, when ^{59}Fe was added to human milk, disproportionate labeling of lactoferrin was obtained; about 80% of the radiolabel was bound to lactoferrin. This was after 1 h of incubation and it appeared that longer incubation would be needed for attempting to reach equilibrium. We have recently shown that after 72 h of incubation at 4°C, isotope distribution in human milk, cow's milk, and formula is similar to that of native iron.[86] As discussed previously with regard to the compartmentalization of iron in human milk, iron in fat globule membranes and casein micelles may not be easily accessible for equilibrium reactions, therefore making lactoferrin the only rapidly available compartment (and one with very high affinity for iron). If this is correct, previous studies using extrinsic labeling may have estimated iron bioavailability from lactoferrin rather than from human milk. Lactoferrin has been shown to survive passage through the infant's gastrointestinal tract and is found intact in the feces of the infant (see below); therefore, lactoferrin also may retain the extrinsic label.

C. MECHANISMS OF IRON ABSORPTION IN INFANTS

Hematological indices for breast-fed infants and the radioisotope absorption studies together speak for a high bioavailability of human milk iron. The question then arises: what mechanism(s) is responsible for this high degree of absorption of iron from human milk? Several possible factors that would influence absorption of iron can be suggested: (1) human milk contains an iron-binding protein, lactoferrin, that may facilitate iron absorption; (2) human milk is low in casein, a protein that may inhibit iron absorption; (3) human milk is lower in protein and protein level in the diet has been negatively correlated to iron absorption; (4) human milk has a high concentration of lactose, a carbohydrate known to enhance iron absorption; or (5) human milk has a conditioning effect on the intestinal mucosa (such as enhanced mucosal growth) which facilitates iron absorption. Of course, the difference in iron bioavailability observed between human milk and cow's milk may be due to several or all of these factors acting synergistically.

An obvious potential candidate for a specific role in iron absorption from human milk is lactoferrin. de Vet and van Gool[87] addressed this possibility, but found that duodenally infused lactoferrin in human adults decreased iron absorption as measured by plasma uptake. The plasma uptake method, however, does not necessarily measure absorption and their data need to be considered with caution. Cox et al.[88] described a putative intestinal receptor in human adults and visualized it by an immunochemical staining method. These authors, however, suggested that lactoferrin inhibits iron absorption and protects the mucosa from iron overload. Their hypothesis was subsequently revised and expanded by Brock[89] who suggested that in early infancy, when iron requirement is low and protein digestion not fully developed, lactoferrin binds iron and is excreted undigested thereby protecting against too large of an iron accumulation at a period of low need for iron. Later in infancy, the proteolytic activity of the infant's gut is increased and lactoferrin can be degraded and the bound iron released and absorbed. McMillan et al.[90] attempted to assess iron absorption from lactoferrin by adding this protein to infant formula and measuring iron absorption in human adults. They added human lactoferrin to a "simulated human milk", having similar concentrations of protein (bovine skim milk and whey), fat, carbohydrate, total minerals, calcium, and phosphorus, and measured incorporation of ^{59}Fe 14 d postingestion. Iron absorption from the "simulated human milk" was 9% and from the same formula with added lactoferrin, 4.7%. Boiled human milk was compared to unboiled milk and the results for iron absorption were similar. These authors, therefore, suggested that lactoferrin is not responsible for the high degree of iron absorption from human milk. Some of the details of their experimental design, however, require further scrutiny. First, the iron content of the "simulated human milk" was three times higher than that of the formula without this protein. McMillan et al.[62] in their previous study showed a strong negative effect of doubling the iron concentration of formula on iron absorption. Second, the method used to saturate lactoferrin and experiments to assure proper saturation were not given in the paper. Iron uptake by lactoferrin can sometimes be slow, despite its high affinity for iron, and is dependent on factors such as pH, anion concentration, and chelators. It has been shown that saturation of pure lactoferrin with iron added as ferrous sulfate is not complete at 24 h.[91] Therefore, if lactoferrin saturation is not assessed, it is quite possible that iron may be present in an inorganic form and possibly become associated to other milk ligands. That this may have been the case in the study by McMillan et al.[90] is indicated by the very high iron to lactoferrin ratio used for the preparation of lactoferrin to be added, namely 200:1 iron to lactoferrin instead of the stoichiometric 2:1 ratio. Taking these observations into account, the experiments of McMillan et al. should not be used as evidence against a role for lactoferrin in iron absorption in infants.

Experiments in animals show conflicting results for the role of lactoferrin in iron absorption. DeLaey et al.[92] used an *in vitro* inverted gut sac system and showed that in rats and guinea pigs, apo-lactoferrin inhibits mucosal iron uptake. Iron-saturated lactoferrin did not have any effect and addition of an antibody to lactoferrin increased iron absorption. In contrast, Fransson et al.[93] demonstrated a more rapid uptake of iron into blood of suckling pigs when ^{59}Fe-lactoferrin was given in a milk formula as compared to ^{59}Fe-labeled ferrous sulfate (Figure 7).

Recently, we have demonstrated the presence of a receptor for lactoferrin in the brush border membrane of infant Rhesus monkeys.[94] We had previously isolated and characterized monkey milk lactoferrin and found it to be very similar to human lactoferrin with regard to molecular weight, amino acid composition, N-terminal sequence, and glycan monosaccharide composition.[59] Similarity was also shown by the cross-reaction between antibody from one species with antigen from the other. Subsequently, we have characterized the receptor with regard to kinetics of iron binding, ontogeny, and dependency on glycan composition.[95,96] The binding of lactoferrin to the receptor was saturable and specific; human transferrin or bovine lactoferrin did not bind at all. The receptor is expressed from fetal life through adulthood with similar affinity toward lactoferrin, but the number of binding sites is highest during infancy. The binding constant for lactoferrin, $K_d = 1.6 \times 10^{-6}\ M$, is similar to that found for transferrin binding to its receptor and of a magnitude compatible with the lactoferrin concentration in the gut. Binding of lactoferrin to its receptor was significantly reduced by removal of terminal fucose residues (with fucosidase) and by the addition of excess fucoidin (a fucose sulfate polymer), strongly implying a functional role for fucose

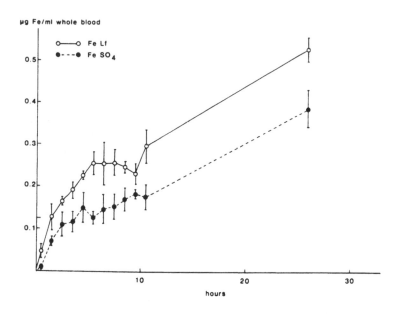

FIGURE 7.   Uptake of ⁵⁹Fe into whole blood of suckling piglets fed ⁵⁹Fe-lac-
toferrin or ⁵⁹FeSO₄.[93]

in the receptor binding of lactoferrin. This would explain why bovine lactoferrin does not
bind to the receptor, since this protein does not have fucose in its glycan moieties.[9] Some
support for fucose being involved in lactoferrin binding to biological membranes can also
be obtained from Spik et al.[9] who found that fucosylated BSA could inhibit binding of
human lactoferrin to macrophages. Mazurier et al.[97] have also recently shown a specific
receptor for lactoferrin in rabbit brush border membranes. They demonstrated specific binding
and visualized the receptor by a ligand-blotting technique. These reports strongly support a
role for lactoferrin in receptor-mediated uptake of iron. The inability of bovine lactoferrin
to bind to the receptor for monkey (or human) lactoferrin, suggests that this mechanism
requires homologous lactoferrin or from a closely related species. This may explain why
Fairweather-Tait et al.[82] found similar iron absorption from formula with ⁵⁸Fe-labeled bovine
lactoferrin and ⁵⁹Fe-labeled ferric chloride. However, it is also possible that ⁵⁸Fe from ferric
chloride was in part bound to lactoferrin in the formula, making the diets more similarly
labeled and only differing in lactoferrin concentration. Alternatively, as the authors suggest,
⁵⁸Fe from lactoferrin may have been dissociated by the lower pH in the gut and may not
have recombined in the small intestine. These methodological considerations emphasize the
difficulties involved in studying iron absorption in infants.

Besides its possible role as a promoter of iron absorption in infants, lactoferrin has also
been suggested to have two other physiological roles. Bullen et al.[98] and Arnold et al.[99]
demonstrated that apo-lactoferrin is bacteriostatic *in vivo* and that addition of iron can abolish
this effect. Thus, it is possible that lactoferrin, which occurs in human milk in a very
unsaturated form,[3] can have a bacteriostatic effect in breast-fed infants. So far, *in vivo*
evidence is lacking, but it is feasible that an inhibitory effect of lactoferrin on the growth
of pathogens can contribute to the lower incidence of infections in breast-fed infants as
compared to formula-fed infants.[100] Another possible effect of lactoferrin is that it may act
as a growth stimulator on the mucosal epithelial cells. Nichols et al.[101] recently showed that
lactoferrin stimulates the incorporation of labeled thymidine in isolated rat crypt cells,
suggesting that lactoferrin may have a proliferative effect on the small intestinal mucosa.
Further studies are needed to evaluate this potential activity in human cell lines.

For all the suggested biological activities, it is necessary that lactoferrin maintains its structure within the gastrointestinal tract of the human infant. Brock et al.[102] showed that lactoferrin is remarkably resistant against proteolysis by trypsin. This may be especially relevant in the infant that has a relatively high gut pH, limiting pepsin activity. Spik et al.[103] found that lactoferrin added to infant formula could be found intact in the stool of these infants. Recently, it was demonstrated that breast-fed infants excrete small but significant quantities of intact lactoferrin in their feces.[104,105] It has also been shown that limited proteolysis of lactoferrin can yield large iron-binding fragments[106] and that these fragments also can donate iron to brush border membranes.[107] Thus, it appears possible that some lactoferrin can survive digestion intact or only be digested to a limited extent and therefore may exert its function in the gut.

V. CONCLUSIONS

Our knowledge of the biochemical nature of iron in milk and formulas has been advanced during the last decade. Unfortunately, our ability to follow the fate of iron provided by these diets in different forms has not kept pace. It seems reasonable to pursue studies on the effect of each individual factor of these infants diets prior to evaluating the net effect of all these together. However, these studies are accompanied with several methodological problems, each of which needs to be taken into account prior to designing the experiment. One may hope that better characterization of diets and the labeled components studied, followed by carefully designed animal studies in appropriate species as well as the use of stable isotopes in human infants will further increase our knowledge of milk iron utilization in infants.

REFERENCES

1. **Masson, P.,** *La Lactoferrine,* Editions Arscia, Bruselles, Belgium, 1970, 232.
2. **Fransson, G.-B. and Lönnerdal, B.,** Iron in human milk, *J. Pediatr.,* 96, 380, 1980.
3. **Schäfer, K. H., Breyer, A. M., and Karte, M.,** Das Spurenelement Eisen in Milch und Milchmischungen, *Z. Kinderheilkd.,* 76, 501, 1955.
4. **Fransson, G.-B. and Lönnerdal, B.,** Distribution of trace elements and minerals in human and cow's milk, *Pediatr. Res.,* 17, 912, 1983.
5. **Lönnerdal, B.,** Iron in breast milk, in *Iron Nutrition in Infancy and Childhood,* Stekel, A., Ed., Nestle, Vevey and Raven Press, New York, 1984, 95.
6. **Metz-Boutique, M.-H., Jolles, J., Mazurier, J., Schoentgen, F., Legrand, D., Spik, G., Montreuil, J., and Jolles, P.,** Human lactotransferrin: amino acid sequence and structural comparisons with other transferrins, *Eur. J. Biochem.,* 145, 659, 1984.
7. **Aisen, P. and Listowski, I.,** Iron transport and storage proteins, *Annu. Rev. Biochem.,* 49, 357, 1980.
8. **Spik, G., Strecker, G., Fournet, B., Bouquelet, S., and Montreuil, J.,** Primary structure of the glycans from human lactotransferrin, *Eur. J. Biochem.,* 121, 413, 1982.
9. **Spik, G., Coddeville, B., Legrand, D., Mazurier, J., Leger, D., Goavec, M., and Montreuil, J.,** A comparative study of the primary structure of glycans from various sero-, lacto- and ovotransferrins. Role of human lactotransferrin glycans, in *Proteins of Iron Storage and Transport,* Spik, G., Montreuil, J., Chrichton, R. R., and Mazurier, J., Eds., Elsevier, Amsterdam, 1985, 47.
10. **Lönnerdal, B.,** Effect of maternal iron status on iron in human milk, in *Human Lactation 2: Maternal and Environmental Factors,* Hamosh, M. and Goldman, A. S., Eds., Plenum Press, New York, 1986, 363.
11. **Prentice, A., Prentice, A. M., Cole, T. J., and Whitehead, R. G.,** Determinants of variations in breast milk protective factor concentrations of rural Gambian mothers, *Arch. Dis. Child.,* 58, 518, 1983.
12. **Houghton, M. R., Gracey, M., Burke, V., Bottrell, C., and Spargo, R. M.,** Breast milk lactoferrin levels in relation to maternal nutritional status, *J. Pediatr. Gastroenterol. Nutr.,* 4, 230, 1985.
13. **Fransson, G.-B., Agarwal, K. N., Gebre-Medhin, M., and Hambraeus, L.,** Increased breast milk iron in severe maternal anemia: physiological "trapping" or leakage?, *Acta Paediatr. Scand.,* 74, 290, 1985.

14. **Sullivan, C. H., Mather, I. H., Greenwalt, D. E., and Madara, P. J.,** Purification of xanthine oxidase from the fat-globule membrane of bovine milk by electrofocusing, *Mol. Cell. Biochem.*, 44, 13, 1982.

15. **Fransson, G.-B. and Lönnerdal, B.,** Iron, zinc, copper and manganese in human milk fat, *Am. J. Clin. Nutr.*, 39, 185, 1984.

16. **Picciano, M. F.,** Mineral content of human milk during a single nursing, *Nutr. Rep. Int.*, 18, 5, 1978.

17. **Forsum, E. and Lönnerdal, B.,** Variation in the contents of nutrients of breast milk during one feeding, *Nutr. Rep. Int.*, 19, 815, 1979.

18. **Bruder, G., Heid, H., Jarasch, E.-D., Keenan, T. W., and Mather, I. H.,** Characteristics of membrane-bound and soluble forms of xanthine oxidase from milk and endothelial cells of capillaries, *Biochim. Biophys. Acta*, 701, 357, 1982.

19. **Van der Westhuyzen, J., van Tonder, S. V., and Fernandes-Costa, F. J.,** Ferritin in breast milk of black urban and rural mothers, *Int. J. Vit. Nutr. Res.*, 56, 287, 1986.

20. **Arosio, P., Ponzone, A., Ferrero, R., Renoldi, I., and Levi, S.,** Characteristics of ferritins in human milk secretions: similarities to serum and tissue ferritins, *Clin. Chim. Acta*, 161, 201, 1986.

21. **Lönnerdal, B., Stanislowski, A. G., and Hurley, L. S.,** Isolation of a low molecular weight zinc binding ligand from human milk, *J. Inorg. Biochem.*, 12, 71, 1980.

22. **Morley, C. G. D. and Bezkorovainy, A.,** Identification of the iron chelate in hepatocyte cytosol, *IRCS Med. Sci.*, 11, 1106, 1983.

23. **Mulligan, M., Althaus, B., and Linder, M. C.,** Non-ferritin, non-heme iron pools in rat tissues, *Int. J. Biochem.*, 18, 791, 1986.

24. **Siimes, M. A., Vuori, E., and Kuitunen, P.,** Breast milk iron: a declining concentration during the course of lactation, *Acta Paediatr. Scand.*, 68, 29, 1979.

25. **Vaughan, L. A., Weber, C. W., and Kemberling, S. R.,** Longitudinal changes in the mineral content of human milk, *Am. J. Clin. Nutr.*, 32, 2301, 1979.

26. **Dewey, K. and Lönnerdal, B.,** Milk and nutrient intake of breast-fed infants from one to six months: relation to growth and fatness, *J. Pediatr. Gastroenterol. Nutr.*, 2, 497, 1983.

27. **Palma, P. A., Seifert, W. E., Caprioli, R. M., and Howell, R. R.,** X-ray fluorescence spectrometry in the analysis of trace elements in human milk, *J. Lab. Clin. Med.*, 102, 88, 1983.

28. **Finley, D. A., Lönnerdal, B., Dewey, K. G., and Grivetti, L. E.,** Inorganic constituents of breast milk from vegetarians and nonvegetarians: relationships with each other and with organic constituents, *J. Nutr.*, 115, 772, 1985.

29. **Murray, M. J., Murray, A. B., Murray, N. J., and Murray, M. B.,** The effect of iron status of Nigerian mothers on that of infants at birth and 6 months, and on the concentration of Fe in breast milk, *Br. J. Nutr.*, 39, 627, 1978.

30. **Feeley, R. M., Eitenmiller, R. R., Jones, J. B., Jr., and Barnhart, H.,** Copper, iron and zinc contents of human milk and early stages of lactation, *Am. J. Clin. Nutr.*, 37, 443, 1983.

31. **Lönnerdal, B., Forsum, E., and Hambraeus, L.,** A longitudinal study of the protein, nitrogen and lactose contents of human milk from Swedish well-nourished mothers, *Am. J. Clin. Nutr.*, 29, 1127, 1976.

32. **Morriss, F. H., Jr., Brewer, E. D., Spedale, S. B., Riddle, L., Temple, D. M., Caprioli, R. M., and West, M. S.,** Relationship of human milk pH during course of lactation to concentrations of citrate and fatty acids, *Pediatrics*, 78, 458, 1986.

33. **Florentino, R. F. and Guirriec, R. M.,** Prevalence of nutritional anemia in infancy and childhood with emphasis on developing countries, in *Iron Nutrition in Infancy and Childhood*, Stekel, A., Ed., Nestle, Vevey and Raven Press, New York, 1984, 61.

34. **Dallman, P. R., Siimes, M. A., and Stekel, A.,** Iron deficiency in infancy and childhood, *Am. J. Clin. Nutr.*, 33, 86, 1980.

35. **Picciano, M. F. and Guthrie, H. A.,** Copper, iron, and zinc contents of mature human milk, *Am. J. Clin. Nutr.*, 29, 242, 1976.

36. **Karmarkar, M. G. and Ramakrishnan, C. V.,** Studies on human lactation. Relation between the dietary intake of lactating women and the chemical composition of milk with regard to principal and certain inorganic constituents, *Acta Pediatr.*, 49, 599, 1960.

37. **Vuori, E., Makinen, S. M., Kara, R., and Kuitunen, P.,** The effects of the dietary intakes of copper, iron, manganese and zinc on the trace element content of human milk, *Am. J. Clin. Nutr.*, 33, 227, 1980.

38. **Fransson, G.-B., Gebre-Medhin, M., and Hambraeus, L.,** The human milk contents of iron, copper, zinc, calcium and magnesium in a population with a habitually high intake of iron, *Acta Paediatr. Scand.*, 73, 471, 1984.

39. **Hallberg, L., Björn-Rasmussen, E., Rossander, L., Suwanik, R., Pleehachinda, R., and Tuntawiroon, M.,** Iron absorption from some Asian meals containing contamination iron, *Am. J. Clin. Nutr.*, 37, 272, 1983.

40. **Moutafchiev, D. A., Shishera, A. C., and Sirakov, L. M.,** Binding of transferrin-iron to the plasma membrane of a lactating rabbit mammary gland cell, *Int. J. Biochem.*, 15, 755, 1983.

41. **Sigman, M. and Lönnerdal, B.,** Identification of a transferrin-receptor mediating iron uptake into rat mammary tissue plasma membranes, *Fed. Proc.,* 46, 438, 1987.

42. **Celada, A., Brusset, R., Gutierrez, J., and Herreros, V.,** No correlation between iron concentration in breast milk and maternal iron stores, *Helv. Paediatr. Acta,* 37, 11, 1982.

43. **Ezekiel, E. and Morgan, E. H.,** Milk iron and its metabolism in the lactating rat, *J. Physiol.,* 165, 336, 1963.

44. **Keen, C. L., Lönnerdal, B., Sloan, M. V., and Hurley, L. S.,** Effect of dietary iron, copper, and zinc chelates of nitrilotriacetic acid (NTA) on trace metal concentrations in rat milk and maternal and pup tissues, *J. Nutr.,* 110, 897, 1980.

45. **Anaokar, S. G. and Garry, P. G.,** Effects of maternal iron nutrition during lactation on milk iron and rat neonatal iron status, *Am. J. Clin. Nutr.,* 34, 1505, 1981.

46. **Sherman, A. R., Guthrie, H. A., Wolinsky, I., and Zulak, I. M.,** Iron deficiency hyperlipidemia in 18-day-old rat pups: effects on milk lipids, lipoprotein lipase, and triglyceride synthesis, *J. Nutr.,* 108, 152, 1978.

47. **Lönnerdal, B., Keen, C. L., and Hurley, L. S.,** Trace elements in milk from various species, in *Trace Element Metabolism in Man and Animals (TEMA) - 4,* Howell, J., McC., Gawthorne, J. M., and White, C. L., Eds., Griffen Press, Netly, South Australia, 1981, 249.

48. **Richardson, T. and Guss, P. S.,** Lipids and metals in fat globule membrane fractions, *J. Dairy Sci.,* 48, 523, 1965.

49. **Hegenauer, J., Saltman, P., Ludwig, D., Ripley, L., and Ley, A.,** Iron-supplemented cow milk. Identification and spectral properties of iron bound to casein micelles, *J. Agric. Food Chem.,* 27, 1294, 1979.

50. **Keen, C. L., Lönnerdal, B., Clegg, M. S., and Hurley, L. S.,** Developmental changes in composition of rat milk: trace elements, minerals, protein, carbohydrate and fat, *J. Nutr.,* 111, 226, 1981.

51. **Lönnerdal, B., Keen, C. L., and Hurley, L. S.,** Iron, copper, zinc and manganese in milk, *Annu. Rev. Nutr.,* 1, 149, 1981.

52. **Lönnerdal, B., Keen, C. L., Hurley, L. S., and Fisher, G. L.,** Developmental changes in the composition of beagle dog milk, *Am. J. Vet. Res.,* 42, 662, 1981.

53. **Keen, C. L., Lönnerdal, B., Clegg, M. S., Hurley, L. S., Morris, J. G., Rogers, Q. R., and Rucker, R. B.,** Developmental changes in composition of cats' milk: trace elements, minerals, protein, carbohydrate and fat, *J. Nutr.,* 112, 1763, 1982.

54. **Jenness, R. and Sloan, R. E.,** The composition of milks of various species: a review, *Dairy Sci. Abstr.,* 32, 599, 1970.

55. **Masson, P. L. and Heremans, J. F.,** Lactoferrin in milk from different species, *Comp. Biochem. Physiol.,* 39B, 119, 1971.

56. **Jordan, S. M. and Morgan, E. H.,** Albumin, transferrin and gammaglobulin metabolism during lactation in the rat, *Q. J. Exp. Physiol.,* 52, 422, 1967.

57. **Leclercq, Y., Sawatzki, G., Wieruszeski, M., Montreuil, J., and Spik, G.,** Primary structure of the glycans from mouse serum and milk transferrins, *Biochem. J.,* 247, 571, 1987.

58. **Elliot, J. I., Senft, B., Erhardt, G., and Fraser, D.,** Isolation of lactoferrin and its concentration in sow's colostrum and milk during a 21-day lactation, *J. Anim. Sci.,* 59, 1080, 1984.

59. **Davidson, L. A. and Lönnerdal, B.,** Isolation and characterization of Rhesus monkey milk lactoferrin, *Pediatr. Res.,* 20, 197, 1986.

60. **Rao, B. S. N., Prasad, J. S., and Sarathy, C. V.,** An animal model to study iron availability from human diets, *Br. J. Nutr.,* 37, 451, 1977.

61. **MacKay, H. M. M.,** Anemia in infancy: its prevalency and prevention, *Arch. Dis. Child.,* 3, 1175, 1928.

62. **McMillan, J. A., Landaw, S. A., and Oski, F. A.,** Iron sufficiency in breast-fed infants and the availability of iron from human milk, *Pediatrics,* 58, 686, 1976.

63. **Saarinen, U. M.,** Need for iron supplementation in infants on prolonged breast-feeding, *J. Pediatr.,* 93, 177, 178.

64. **Oski, F. A. and Landaw, S. A.,** Inhibition of iron absorption from human milk by baby food, *Am. J. Dis. Child.,* 134, 459, 1980.

65. **Picciano, M. F. and Deering, R. H.,** The influence of feeding regimens on iron status during infancy, *Am. J. Clin. Nutr.,* 33, 746, 1980.

66. **Siimes, M. A., Salmenperä, L., and Perheentupa, J.,** Exclusive breast-feeding for 9 months: risk of iron deficiency, *J. Pediatr.,* 104, 196, 1984.

67. **Duncan, B., Schifman, R. B., Corrigan, J. J., and Schaefer, C.,** Iron and the exclusively breast-fed infant from birth to six months, *J. Pediatr. Gastroenterol. Nutr.,* 4, 421, 1985.

68. **Iwai, Y., Takanashi, T., Nakao, Y., and Mikawa, H.,** Iron status of low birth weight infants on breast and formula feeding, *Eur. J. Pediatr.,* 145, 63, 1986.

69. **Reeves, J. D., Yip, R., Kyley, V. A., and Dallman, P. R.,** Iron deficiency in infants: the influence of mild antecedent infection, *J. Pediatr.,* 105, 874, 1985.

70. **Fomon, S. J. and Strauss, R. G.**, Nutrient deficiencies in breast-fed infants, *N. Engl. J. Med.*, 299, 355, 1978.

71. **Saarinen, U. M. and Siimes, M. A.**, Iron absorption from breast milk, cow's milk, and iron-supplemented formula: an opportunistic use of changes in total body iron determined by hemoglobin, ferritin, and body weight in 132 infants, *Pediatr. Res.*, 13, 143, 1979.

72. **Garry, P. J., Owen, G. M., Hooper, E. M., and Gilbert, B. A.**, Iron absorption from human milk and formula with and without iron supplementation, *Pediatr. Res.*, 15, 822, 1981.

73. **Fomon, S. J.**, Absorption of iron calculated from estimated changes in total body iron (Letter), *Pediatr. Res.*, 16, 161, 1982.

74. **Schulz, J. and Smith, N. J.**, A quantitative study of the absorption of food iron in infants and children, *J. Dis. Child.*, 95, 109, 1958.

75. **Hallberg, L.**, Bioavailability of dietary iron in man, *Annu. Rev. Nutr.*, 1, 123, 1981.

76. **Garby, L. and Sjölin, S.**, Absorption of labelled iron in infants less than three months old, *Acta Paediatr.*, 48(Suppl. 117), 24, 1959.

77. **Heinrich, H. C., Gabbe, E. E., Whang, D. H., Bender-Götze, Ch., and Schäfer, K. H.**, Ferrous and hemoglobin $^{-59}$Fe absorption from supplemented cow milk in infants with normal and depleted iron stores, *Z. Kinderheilkd.*, 120, 251, 1975.

78. **Saarinen, U. M., Siimes, M. A., and Dallman, P. R.**, Iron absorption in infants: high bioavailability of breast milk iron as indicated by the extrinsic tag method of iron absorption and by the concentration of serum ferritin, *J. Pediatr.*, 91, 36, 1977.

79. **Llanes, T. E. and Lönnerdal, B.**, Digestibility of human, bovine and Rhesus monkey milk, *Fed. Proc.*, 46, 895, 1987.

80. **Janghorbani, M., Ting, B. T. G., and Fomon, S. J.**, Erythrocyte incorporation of ingested stable isotope of iron (^{58}Fe), *Am. J. Hematol.*, 21, 277, 1986.

81. **Saarinen, U. M. and Siimes, M. A.**, Iron absorption from infant milk formula and the optimal level of iron supplementation, *Acta Paediatr. Scand.*, 66, 719, 1977.

82. **Fairweather-Tait, S. J., Balmer, S. E., Scott, P. H., and Minski, M. J.**, Lactoferrin and iron absorption in newborn infants, *Pediatr. Res.*, 22, 651, 1987.

83. **Björn-Rasmussen, E., Hallberg, L., and Walker, R. B.**, Food iron absorption in man. II. Isotopic exchange of iron between labeled foods and between a food and an iron salt, *Am. J. Clin. Nutr.*, 26, 1311, 1973.

84. **Fomon, S. J.**, *Infant Nutrition*, W. B. Saunders, Philadelphia, 1974, 575.

85. **Fransson, G.-B. and Lönnerdal, B.**, Distribution of added ^{59}Fe among different fractions of human and cow's milk, *Näringsforskringr*, 27, 108, 1983.

86. **Davidson, L. A. and Lönnerdal, B.**, Iron absorption from human milk and infant formula using the nursing Rhesus monkey as a model, submitted.

87. **de Vet, B. J. C. M. and van Gool, J.**, Lactoferrin and iron absorption in the small intestine, *Acta Med. Scand.*, 196, 393, 1974.

88. **Cox, T. M., Mazurier, J., Spik, G., Montreuil, J., and Peters, T. J.**, Iron binding proteins and influx of iron across the duodenal brush border, *Biochim. Biophys. Acta*, 588, 120, 1979.

89. **Brock, J. H.**, Lactoferrin in human milk: its role in iron absorption and protection against enteric infection in the newborn infant, *Arch. Dis. Child.*, 55, 417, 1980.

90. **McMillan, J. A., Oski, F. A., Lourie, G., Tomarelli, R. M., and Landaw, S. A.**, Iron absorption from human milk, simulated human milk, and proprietary formulas, *Pediatrics*, 60, 896, 1977.

91. **Bates, G. W., Billups, C., and Saltman, P.**, The kinetics and mechanism of iron(III) exchange between chelates and transferrin. I. The complexes of citrate and nitrilotriacetic acid, *J. Biol. Chem.*, 242, 2810, 1967.

92. **DeLaey, P., Masson, P. L., and Heremans, J. F.**, The role of lactoferrin in iron absorption, *Protides Biol. Fluids*, 16, 627, 1968.

93. **Fransson, G.-B., Thoren-Tolling, K., Jones, B., Hambraeus, L., and Lönnerdal, B.**, Absorption of lactoferrin-iron in suckling pigs, *Nutr. Res.*, 3, 373, 1983.

94. **Davidson, L. A. and Lönnerdal, B.**, Isolation and characterization of monkey milk lactoferrin and its brush border receptor, *Fed. Proc.*, 43, 468, 1984.

95. **Davidson, L. A. and Lönnerdal, B.**, Isolation and characterization of monkey milk lactoferrin and identification of a specific brush border receptor, in *Proteins of Iron Metabolism*, Spik, G. et al., Eds., Elsevier, Amsterdam, 1985, 275.

96. **Davidson, L. A. and Lönnerdal, B.**, Specific binding of lactoferrin to brush border membrane: ontogeny and effect of glycan chain, *Am. J. Physiol.*, 254, G580, 1988.

97. **Mazurier, J., Montreuil, J., and Spik, G.**, Visualization of lactotransferrin brush-border membrane receptors by ligand-blotting, *Biochim. Biophys. Acta*, 821, 453, 1985.

98. **Bullen, J. J., Rogers, H. J., and Leigh, L.**, Iron-binding proteins in human milk and resistance to *Escherichia coli* infection in infants, *Br. J. Med.*, 1, 69, 1972.

99. **Arnold, R. R., Cole, M. F., and McGhee, J. R.,** A bactericidal effect for human milk lactoferrin, *Science,* 197, 263, 1977.

100. Committee on Nutrition, Relationship between iron status and incidence of infection in infancy, *Pediatrics,* 62, 246, 1978.

101. **Nichols, B. L., McKeen, K. S., Henry, J. F., and Putnam, M.,** Human lactoferrin stimulates thymidine incorporation into DNA of rat crypt cells, *Pediatr. Res.,* 21, 563, 1987.

102. **Brock, J. H., Arzabe, F., Lampreave, F., and Pineiro, A.,** The effect of trypsin on bovine transferrin and lactoferrin, *Biochim. Biophys. Acta,* 446, 214, 1976.

103. **Spik, G., Brunet, B., Mazurier-Dehaine, C., Fontaine, G., and Montreuil, J.,** Characterization and properties of the human and bovine lactotransferrins extracted from the feces of newborn infants, *Acta Paediatr. Scand.,* 71, 979, 1982.

104. **Prentice, A., Ewing, G., Roberts, S. B., Lucas, A., MacCarthy, A., Jarjou, L. M. A., and Whitehead, R. G.,** The nutritional role of breast milk IgA and lactoferrin, *Acta Paediatr. Scand.,* 76, 592, 1987.

105. **Davidson, L. A. and Lönnerdal, B.,** Persistence of human milk proteins in the breast-fed infant, *Acta Paediatr. Scand.,* 76, 733, 1987.

106. **Legrand, D., Mazurier, J., Aubert, J.-P., Loucheux-Lefebvre, M.-H., Montreuil, J., and Spik, G.,** Evidence for interactions between the 30kDa N- and 50kDa C-terminal tryptic fragments of human lactotransferrin, *Biochem. J.,* 236, 839, 1986.

107. **Davidson, L. A. and Lönnerdal, B.,** Interaction of various forms of lactoferrin with brush border membranes from the Rhesus monkey, *FASEB J.,* 2, A652, 1988.

Chapter 6

IRON IN FORMULAS AND BABY FOODS

Sean R. Lynch and Richard F. Hurrell

TABLE OF CONTENTS

I. INTRODUCTION

Full term infants are born with sufficient iron to supply the physiological needs of the first 2 months of extrauterine life;[1] 75% is in circulating hemoglobin. With the physiological postnatal fall in hemoglobin concentration, this iron is redistributed to storage sites. However, owing to rapid growth, the reserve is essentially depleted by 4 months of age. Between 4 and 12 months, the infant becomes dependent on an adequate and continuous supply of exogenous iron. Based on estimates published by Smith and Rios,[2] Stekel[3] calculated an average daily requirement of 0.49 mg for the first 6 months and 0.90 mg between the ages of 6 and 12 months in nonbreast-fed infants. Thus, at 1 year of age, absorbed iron contributes 30% of the daily hemoglobin iron turnover. By comparison, an adult man meets only 5% of these needs through absorption.[1]

Although such estimates underline the importance of the dietary iron supply in infancy, it is noteworthy that iron losses account for 40 to 50% of the calculated requirement. Estimates of iron loss are based on the measurement of [51]chromium-labeled red cells in the stools of 2- to 17-month-old infants fed on cow's milk and cereals. In this study, the average daily blood loss was 0.64 ml or 0.22 mg.[4] Values were threefold higher if acute gastroenteritis was present. Similar results have been obtained by other workers in older infants[5,6] and iron losses can be increased markedly if young infants are given fresh milk.[7-9]

Infants fed exclusively on human milk are estimated to have an average daily iron *intake* of only 0.29 mg at 6 months. Nevertheless, the majority of exclusively breast-fed full-term infants are able to maintain an iron status equal to that of controls receiving iron-supplemented formula for 6 to 9 months.[10] This apparent anomaly is largely attributable to the very high bioavailability of the iron in human milk, 45 to 75% being absorbed,[11] although it is evident that iron loss must be minimal in the breast-fed infant and that the latter factor may well play an equally important role in maintaining balance.

II. DETERMINANTS OF IRON ABSORPTION

Human milk possesses properties that promote iron absorption. The factors responsible are poorly understood. It has been proposed that the high concentrations of cysteine, adenine nucleotides, and taurine may play a role;[12] however, recent observations suggest that lactoferrin is the most important factor. It has three properties that together may ensure specific delivery of iron to the mucosal cell. It has a high affinity for iron under the luminal conditions in the duodenum, specific receptors for lactoferrin are present in the mucosal cells of the upper small intestine, and lactoferrin is relatively resistant to digestion by the enzymes secreted into the gut lumen.

In meals consisting of foods other than human milk, factors governing iron availability are much more complex;[13] however, several isotopic investigations in adults have led to a unified concept of the luminal phase of iron absorption that has gained general acceptance. Almost all the iron we ingest appears to enter one of two common pools before being absorbed.[13,14] The smaller pool comprises heme-iron compounds derived from meat and fish. Iron in this form is virtually always highly available. The larger pool is composed of all other forms of food iron as well as any inorganic iron present. This iron is much less bioavailable and its absorption is very dependent on other factors present in the meal. The differences in bioavailability between the two pools are illustrated by a study of the diets of young Swedish men.[14] Iron absorbed from the heme pool provided one third of daily requirements although the pool itself represented only 5% of the dietary iron.

Apart from human milk, the major sources of dietary iron for the infant in industrialized countries, such as the U.S. are iron-fortified formulas and dry infant cereals.[15] The quantity of meat eaten during the first year rarely supplies a large amount of iron. Thus, there is total dependence on dietary non-heme iron during this critical period, making a clear understanding of factors affecting bioavailability especially important. As the diet becomes more varied in the older child, the major sources of iron are meats and iron-fortified cereals.

A. BIOAVAILABILITY OF NONHEME FOOD IRON
1. Measurement of Nonheme Iron Absorption

Iron absorption can be measured in infants and young children by monitoring changes in iron status, chemical iron balance, or the use of radioisotopic methods. The first two techniques are cumbersome and time consuming. Moreover, while the results may be the most direct measures of iron assimilation, they lack precision. Most reliable information has been derived from radioiron studies. However, this method is also subject to considerable variability when different subjects are compared or even when measurements are made in the same subject on different days.[16]

The early studies of foods that were biosynthetically labeled with radioactive iron established a firm scientific basis for the method.[17] Plant foods were grown in hydroponic media containing radioiron and animal foods were prepared from animals injected with the appropriate radioisotope.

Iron absorption can be measured by whole body counting, the calculation of radioisotopic balance, or the measurement of the red cell utilization of radioactive iron.[13] The convenience and sensitivity of measuring red cell utilization has made it the most popular method for studies of iron bioavailability involving normal individuals and otherwise healthy people with iron deficiency.

Biosynthetically labeled foods yielded important information; however, as indicated earlier, it soon became apparent that the bioavailability of iron in different foods depended not only on the properties of the food item itself, but also on the other components of the meal in which it was eaten. Fortunately the crucial observations of Cook et al.[18] and Björn-Rasmussen et al.[19] provided the basis of the current simplified method for measuring percentage iron absorption from a meal with several food items. They studied complex meals and demonstrated that virtually all the food iron other than heme behaves in terms of absorption as though it is present in a common iron pool that can be tagged by the mere mixing of a small amount of a soluble radioactive iron salt, such as ferric chloride or ferrous sulfate with a major component of the meal (extrinsic tag). The common pool concept has not been documented for all possible food iron sources, but numerous studies have confirmed the original observations. There are only a few known exceptions. Complete equilibration may not occur with whole rice grains,[20] the iron storage compounds ferritin and hemosiderin,[21] and some poorly soluble iron salts, such as sodium iron pyrophosphate and ferric orthophosphate which may contaminate food or be added as an iron supplement.[22,23]

Most studies of food iron bioavailability have been carried out in adults because of the potential dangers of administering radioactive compounds to children. Frequently the individuals studied were iron-replete men whose relative iron requirements are much lower than those of growing children. For this reason, it was necessary to devise a method for comparing measurements in subjects with differing iron needs. The use of a "reference dose" consisting of a freshly prepared solution of 3 mg iron as $FeSO_4$ and sufficient ascorbic acid to provide a 2:1 molar ratio made it possible. Iron in this form is essentially all bioavailable and differences in absorption are only a reflection of the physiological factors that control its assimilation in the individual being studied.[13,24] Average percentage reference dose absorption in iron-deficient children has been established (60%) making it possible to predict bioavailability in iron-deficient infants from studies in adults, by correcting values based on the ratio between the observed percentage absorption of the reference dose and 60%.[24,25] More recently it has become apparent from comparisons between serum ferritin concentrations and reference dose absorption that similar calculations can be based on serum ferritin values.[101]

TABLE 1
Effect of Protein on Non-heme Iron
Availability

Protein	% Absorption
None[a]	44.4
Bovine serum albumin	23.7
Casein	6.2
Egg white	12.2
Wheat gluten	5.2
Whey protein	3.9
Soy protein isolate	1.5

[a]   Data from Reference 27: all values calculated to reflect absorption at a ferritin of 12 $\mu g/l$.

2. Bioavailability of Iron in Baby Foods

The complex nature of the Western diets of adults that characteristically contain appreciable quantities of meat probably ensures adequate iron bioavailability under most circumstances. In infancy, the diet is much simpler. It may comprise only a few food sources with very little or no meat. Financial constraints may also be placed on food choices, particularly in developing countries. The selection of staple can, therefore, have a profound effect on iron bioavailability.

a. Cow's Milk

Milk is often the only source of iron during the first few months of life. It is the major constituent of most infant formula preparations and usually a significant component of the weaning diet. The bioavailability of iron in cow's milk is significantly less than that in human milk. A comparative study in adults demonstrated mean absorptions of 20.8% for human milk and 13.6% for cow's milk.[26] The factors responsible for the superior bioavailability of iron in human milk remain speculative. Iron is absorbed less well from cow's milk even when it is processed to resemble human milk in terms of nutrient composition with respect to protein, fat, carbohydrate, ascorbic acid, calcium, phosphorus, and iron content.[26]

The possible role of the protein component in milk in determining bioavailability has been reexamined recently. Both the casein and the whey protein fractions of cow's milk markedly reduce iron absorption from a meal comprising semipurified ingredients.[27] Absorption was reduced from 44.4% without protein to 6.2 and 3.9% when casein or whey protein, respectively, was included (Table 1). *In vitro* testing suggested that this was a specific protein effect. The dialyzability of the iron present using a modification of the simulated gastric digestion model of Miller et al.[28] was measured. Both protein fractions reduced the proportion of dialyzable iron, but extensive enzyme hydrolysis of the protein restored dialyzability.

The role of lactoferrin which is present in high concentrations in human milk but not in cow's milk is uncertain. McMillan et al.[26] reported that the addition of a human lactoferrin to cow's milk depressed absorption. However, recent studies in infant Rhesus monkeys by Davidson and Lönnerdal demonstrate that lactoferrin is resistant to proteolysis in the infant gastrointestinal tract and shows specific binding to the brush border of the small intestine, suggesting that it may play an important role in facilitating iron absorption from primate milk.[12]

There is little doubt that iron availability in cow's milk does not match that of human milk, but there do not appear to be major differences when it is compared with other infant foods.[29] In an extensive series of studies designed to evaluate the effect of proteins derived from different sources, bioavailability was reduced by about 50% when milk replaced animal tissue.[30] A similar effect occurred with other dairy products. A recent study[91] of several cow's milk formulas fortified with ferrous sulfate (10 to 19 mg elemental iron per liter) demonstrated that 2.9 to 5.1% of the iron was absorbed by infants aged 5 to 18 months, an amount that was considered insufficient to meet the child's requirements. Absorption from formulas containing at least 100 mg ascorbic acid per liter was 5.9 to 11.3% and they provided sufficient bioavailable iron.

b. Legumes

Soybean products have been used in a wide variety of infant foods and soy-based infant formula is often substituted for milk where possible allergy to cow's milk is encountered. Soybeans and other legumes contain comparatively large quantities of native iron. However, studies of its bioavailability are characterized by the variability of the results reported. Some earlier investigations using biosynthetically labeled beans[31,32] demonstrated relatively high bioavailability with mean absorption values of 11 to 12% in adults. On the other hand, Björn-Rasmussen et al.[33] reported a geometric mean value of only 1.5% for biosynthetically labeled soybeans. The percentage absorption of an extrinsic tag added to each of these meals was 1.7%. Ashworth and March[25] found bioavailability to be low in children. Most recent studies have also demonstrated poor bioavailability,[34,35,90] although Rios et al.[36] reported food iron absorption to be higher from a soy-based than from a milk-based formula in 4- to 7-month-old infants, 5.4 vs. 3.9%.

The reason for the discrepant observations is not known, but it does not appear to be the result of technical flaws or incomplete equilibration of radioiron with the non-heme common pool.[37] The inhibitory effect is preserved in soy protein products[34] and similar percentage iron absorption levels have been observed in meals containing black beans, mung beans, lentils, and split peas.[38] The factors responsible have not been identified. The seed coats of many legumes have a high content of tannin which is known to be a potent inhibitor of iron absorption;[39] however, some beans, such as soybeans and mung beans do not contain significant quantities of tannin. Moreover, the seeds are often dehulled before consumption, thereby reducing the tannin content.

Phytate, which has long been regarded as a possible inhibitor, is found in the cotyledonous fraction of the seeds.[40] For this reason we recently compared iron absorption from biosynthetically labeled soybeans grown by hydroponic culture in nutrient media with low and high phosphate concentrations respectively. A twofold difference in bean phytate and phosphate concentration did not affect absorption.[41]

Recent observations suggest that the inhibitory factors reside in the protein fraction. Extensive hydrolysis of soy protein products with papain markedly reduces their inhibitory effects on iron absorption in adult human volunteers.[27]

c. Cereals

Cereals are important weaning foods, but little new information has become available since their effects on iron absorption were recently extensively reviewed.[37] This subject is therefore, summarized only briefly here. In the International Nutritional Anemia Consultative Group review, the effect of wheat, rice, and maize on iron bioavailability was compared by using published observations. Absorption values from meals in which one cereal made up the bulk of the food eaten were compiled (Table 2). Meals containing a powerful inhibitor or enhancer were excluded. The effect of variations in iron status among the individual studied was removed by expressing all results at a reference dose absorption of 40%. Wheat flour (60 to 80% extraction) was absorbed with a mean corrected percentage absorption value of 30.9%. Comparable values for rice and maize were 6.5 and 3.7%. Sorghum has not been studied as extensively, but availability appears to be even lower.

TABLE 2
Iron Availability in Cereal Meals

Cereal	No. of studies	Weighted mean % absorption (±SD)
Wheat[a]	7	30.9 (±13.3)
Rice	5	6.5 (±4.0)
Maize	7	3.7 (±1.2)
Sorghum[b]	1	3.5

[a]   Data for wheat, rice, and maize from Reference 37.
[b]   Morck, Lynch, Cook, unpublished data, single study
      with 18 observations.

The factors affecting iron absorption from cereals have not been defined with any degree of precision. Phytate, various fiber materials, and polyphenols may all be present and have been suspected of playing a role. Wheat has been studied the most extensively. Bran is known to be the inhibitory component in wheat flour and to reduce iron bioavailability in a dose-dependent fashion.[42,43] Both the phytate and fiber are concentrated in this fraction during milling; however, its inhibitory properties are not modified by degradation of the phytate by endogenous phytases.[43] Moreover, wheat bran and oat bran added to a breakfast meal are equally inhibitory despite a 20-fold difference in phytate-phosphorus content.[37] Finally, monoferric phytate, the major iron form in bran, is well absorbed by dogs.[44]

III. FORMULATION OF FOODS USED IN INFANCY

A. COW'S MILK

Evaporated milk products as well as commercial infant foods based on milk and cereals were developed toward the end of the 19th century. Prior to that time, there was virtually no safe and reliable alternative to breast feeding. For the first half of this century, evaporated milk was the most widely accepted infant food; however, the nutrient composition of cow's milk is not entirely appropriate for the young child. It has far higher quantities of protein and sodium, and a lower calcium to phosphate ratio than does human milk. In addition, the feeding of fresh pasteurized cow's milk in early infancy has been reported to contribute to the development of iron deficiency by inducing intestinal blood loss in some infants.[7-9] Blood loss can be diminished by substituting heat-processed formula for cow's milk or by reducing the amount consumed.

The iron intakes of infants fed a weaning diet based on cow's milk fall short of the Recommended Daily Allowance (RDA) of iron in the U.S. of 15 mg/d.[45] The 24-h dietary intake data from the Second National Health and Nutrition Examination Survey carried out in the U.S. between 1976 and 1980 (NHANES II) revealed iron intakes of 7.8 and 14.9 mg for infants 7 to 12 months of age who were fed mixed diets containing solid foods and either cow's milk or infant formulas, respectively.[46]

In 1983, the Committee on Nutrition of the American Academy of Pediatrics made the following recommendation covering the feeding of cow's milk to infants aged 6 to 12 months:[47]

"If breast-feeding has been completely discontinued and infants are consuming one-third of their calories as supplemental foods consisting of a balanced mixture of cereals, vegetables, fruits and other foods (thereby assuring adequate sources of both iron and vitamin C), whole cow's milk may be introduced. The amount fed should be limited to less than 1 L daily. Most infants who are not breast-fed should be consuming a significant portion of their calories from supplemental foods after they are 6 months old; those who are not should be given iron-fortified formula."

B. INFANT FORMULAS

Infant formulas are manufactured to resemble the nutrient composition of human milk as closely as possible. They are usually based on cow's milk. The first adaptation to be made was the addition of carbohydrate, lactose, sucrose, or maltodextrin, to reduce the concentration of protein, fat, and minerals per unit of energy. The original formulas were also acidified by the addition of lactic or citric acids. Later, biological acidification with lactic acid-producing microorganisms was introduced. The latter formulas have the advantages of a reduced risk of microbial contamination and improved protein digestibility. As a result of the growth of the technology for separating milk components, most adapted formulas are now based on skimmed milk, demineralized whey, vegetable oils, or milk fat and vegetable oil mixtures together with the necessary vitamins and minerals. In the U.S., ready-to-feed formulas are in common use. They may also contain gums and carrageenan to prolong product stability. Elsewhere, spray-dried powders are most widely used.

The incorporation of demineralized whey adds extra lactose to the product and improves its whey protein content. The whey protein to casein ratio of 20:80 normally found in cow's milk is increased to 60:40, similar to that found in human milk,[48] however, it is important to note that whey protein is itself a mixture of proteins. One of the predominant whey proteins of human milk, lactoferrin, is virtually absent from cow's milk. Conversely, β-lactoglobulin, the major whey protein in bovine milk is not found in human milk.[48] The possible importance of lactoferrin to non-heme iron absorption and the inhibitory properties of whey protein and casein in cow's milk have already been described.

Not all milk-based formulas are whey predominant. Casein-predominant formulas based on skim milk are also produced, because they are less expensive. In some infants they may have other advantages, such as better satiety, less regurgitation, and lower allergenicity.

In the U.S., soy formulas make up 10 to 20% of the market.[29] They are rarely used in Europe. Soy protein isolate plus methionine, and glucose or maltodextrin replace milk proteins and lactose, respectively, in these products. They are often prescribed for infants who are allergic or intolerant to milk proteins and can be used in the management of galactosemia.

1. Guidelines and Regulations for Iron Fortification

The nutrient contents of all infant formulas are subject to guidelines and regulations promulgated by several different agencies.[49-54] These recommendations are generally based on the levels of the nutrients found in human milk although, as with iron, poor bioavailability in the formula is taken into account.

The FAO/WHO Codex Alimentarius Commission[51] has issued guidelines for the composition of infant formula. The most recent recommendations in the U.S. were issued in 1983 by the American Academy of Pediatrics.[53] They differ only slightly from their 1976 recommendations[54] which form the basis of the Infant Formula Act passed by the U.S. Congress in 1980. In Europe, the European Economic Community is preparing draft regulations[52] for its 12 member countries that are largely based on guidelines issued by the European Society for Pediatric Gastroenterology and Nutrition (ESPGAN).[49,50] The recommended levels for iron suggested by these different agencies are summarized in Table 3. The recommended levels for calcium, phosphorus, and protein that are potential inhibitors of iron absorption, and vitamin C which is generally enhancing, are also given.

The minimum recommended level for iron ranges from 0.5 to 1.0 mg/100 kcal (3.5 to 7.0 mg/l) and the maximum from 1.5 to 2.5 mg/100 kcal (10.5 to 17.5 mg/l). In noniron fortified formulas, the minimum has been set at 0.15 mg/kcal (about 1 mg/l) which is the quantity of native iron that should be present in the formula. The ESPGAN[49] believed that there was no real justification for the fortification of infant formula with iron before the third month of life, but recommended 1 mg iron per 100 kcal from 3 months onward and

TABLE 3
Guidelines for the Level of Iron and Selected Nutrients per kcal[a] in Infant Formula and a Comparison with Their Respective Levels in Human and Bovine Milk

Agency	Iron (mg) Min	Iron (mg) Max	Protein (g) Min	Protein (g) Max	Calcium (mg) Min	Phosphorus (mg)[b] Min	Phosphorus (mg)[b] Max	Vit D (mg) min	Ref.
Codex Alimentarius	0.15—1.0[c]	—	1.8	4.0	50	25	—	8	51
EEC Draft	0.5	1.5	1.8	3.0	50	25	90	8	52
ESPGAN									
Starting formula	0.15—1.0[c]	—	1.8	2.8	60	30	50	8	49
Follow-up formula	1.0	2.0	3.0	5.5	90	60	—	—	50
AAP/CON	0.15—1.0[c]	2.5[3]	1.8	4.5	60	30	—	8	53
Human milk	0.10	—		1.3	48	22	5.5		48
Bovine milk	0.08	—		5.1	184	146	3.1		48

[a] An infant formula contains about 68 kcal/100 ml.[49]

[b] Ca:P ratio should be 1.2 to 2.0[49] or 1.1 to 2.1.[53]

[c] In an iron-fortified product.

1 to 2 mg/100 kcal in follow-up formula used between 6 and 12 months of age. On the other hand, while recognizing that infants are at greater risk for iron deficiency from 6 to 12 months, the American Academy of Pediatrics Committee on Nutrition (AAP/CON) advised the early use of an iron-fortified formula in an attempt to increase iron stores and prevent iron deficiency.[15]

The protein, calcium, phosphorus, and vitamin C levels in infant formulas (Table 3) recommended by different agencies vary only slightly. The recommendations for the follow-up formula include more protein, calcium, and phosphorus which may be inhibitory to iron absorption. Nevertheless, the ESPGAN[50] did not suggest further nutrient modification since the infant's iron requirements are probably satisfied by the consumption of other weaning foods at this stage.

It is noteworthy that the iron levels in both human and cow's milk are only $\frac{1}{25}$ to $\frac{1}{50}$ those in iron-fortified formulas. Weinberg[55] has expressed the concern that large amounts of unabsorbed iron might stimulate the growth of microorganisms in the intestine and predispose the baby to infections; however, after reviewing the results of various clinical trials, the AAP/CON decided that there was no evidence to justify a change in their recommendations for enriching infant formula with iron.[56] Others have also concluded that the fortification of infant formula with iron does not cause a greater incidence of gastrointestinal symptoms.[57]

2. Iron Content of Commercial Infant Formulas

It is evident that the manufacturers of infant formulas have a relatively wide range of recommended limits for the level of iron in their products. In practice, most iron fortified formulas in the U.S. are designed to contain about 1.7 mg iron per 100 kcal (12 mg/l) and those in Europe 0.7 to 1.2 mg/100 kcal (5 to 8 mg/l). In the follow-up formula, the level is 1.7 mg/100 kcal (12 mg/l). Protein in whey-predominant infant formulas is usually set toward the lower end of the recommended range, about 2.3 g/100 kcal; calcium and phosphorus are often 60 to 100% higher than the minimum given in the guidelines because of the high level of these minerals in cow's milk. Calcium and phosphorus are removed from whey during demineralization. The calcium is added back to the formula to maintain a suitable Ca:P ratio. Ascorbic acid levels are approximately those recommended (8 mg/100 kcal), although most manufacturers add additional quantities to allow for degradation during processing and storage. Soy formulas customarily have a slightly higher protein content (3 g/100 kcal) than milk-based formulas and sometimes a higher concentration of vitamin C, but similar levels of iron, calcium, and phosphorus. Much of the phosphorus is in the form of phytate.

Several workers have measured the actual levels of nutrients including iron in infant formulas purchased commercially.[58-61] In the most recent study, Lönnerdal et al.[61] analyzed 53 formulas collected from the U.S., several European countries, and Japan in 1980. Non-fortified formulas were available in the U.S., West Germany, and Sweden. The level of iron was found to range from 0.17 to 58.5 mg/l. The U.S. formulas had the highest mean iron level. Six formulas purchased had iron concentrations greater than 50 mg/l (7 mg/100 kcal) which is almost three times higher than the suggested maximum value (Table 3). Kirkpatrick et al.[59] analyzed 17 ready-to-feed and powdered formulas in Canada and reported iron levels in the products as consumed from 0.3 to 14 mg/l with a mean value of about 5 mg/l. Most European and Japanese formulas contained 5 to 12 mg/l of fortification iron.

C. INFANT CEREALS

Cereals play an important role in infant feeding and are often the first supplementary foods offered. All grains as well as certain roots (tapioca) and seeds (soybeans and ground nuts) are used in the manufacture of infant cereals. The products may contain one or more cereals with sugar or honey and are often mixed with milk, soybean products, vegetables, or fruit. When intended for young infants, they are processed to facilitate digestion and to allow easy dispersion in water, milk, or juice. Heat or enzymes are employed in this treatment. A complete cereal is fortified with vitamins and minerals and is formulated to supply all the infant's nutrient requirements per unit of energy.

The first infant cereals sold commercially were milk-cereal mixtures. They were marketed in 1867 by Baron von Liebig and in 1868 by Henri Nestle in Germany and Switzerland.[62] It was not until 1933 that the first precooked dry infant cereals were introduced into the U.S. by Mead Johnson.

1. Guidelines and Regulations for Iron Fortification

The composition of infant cereal is regulated less strictly than that of infant formula. The FAO/WHO Codex Alimentarius gives guidelines for the levels of protein and sodium, but makes no recommendations for iron, vitamin C, and other nutrients.[51] The AAP/CON[15] and the ESPGAN[50] guidelines do not agree about the effectiveness of iron-fortified cereals in combatting iron deficiency.

In the U.S., the 1971 Food and Drug Administration Guidelines[63] recommended 47 mg iron per 100 g powder, and this was endorsed by AAP/CON.[15] Infant cereals are an important source of iron for infants aged 7 to 12 months in the U.S.[46] Infant cereals have also been reported to be the major source of iron from the start of the weaning period to about 18 months of age in Canada[64] and have been calculated to provide as much as 80% of the total dietary intake.[59]

The ESPGAN[50] has stated that the addition of iron to infant cereals is not a reliable method of enriching the diet with iron although they do recommend a level of 50 mg/100 g for iron-fortified products. The French Pediatric Society[65] does not recommend the fortification of infant cereals with iron and most infant cereals in France are not fortified.

2. Iron Content of Commercial Infant Cereals

In practice, infant cereal manufacturers in the U.S. and Canada formulate their products to contain about 50 mg of elemental iron per 100 g and similar or slightly higher values have been reported in products purchased commercially for analysis.[59,66] The levels of iron in European infant cereals vary more, but are generally much lower than those in the U.S., presumably a reflection of the ESPGAN[50] guidelines. Cereals often contain about 20 mg iron per 100 g and milk-cereal mixtures usually have 7.5 mg iron per 100 g.

Despite the variation in the levels of iron in North American and European products, it is interesting to note that due to different weaning practices, the total amount of iron contained in a recommended serving size is similar. In the U.S., the recommended serving size for infant cereals is 7 to 14 g.[15] This would provide 23 to 47% of the U.S. RDA for iron in one meal. In Europe, the recommended serving size for an infant over 6 months of age is 25 g for an infant cereal (to be mixed with milk) and 50 g for a milk-cereal mixture. Assuming iron fortification levels of 20 mg and 7.5 mg/100 g, these products provide 33 and 25% of the U.S. RDA for iron, respectively; however, an infant cereal meal in the U.S. clearly provides far less of the infant's total energy intake than is the case in Europe.

D. OTHER COMMERCIALLY PREPARED BABY FOODS

The consumption of other commercially prepared baby foods in industrialized countries is considerable. In the U.S. and Sweden for instance, the average annual consumption is more than 600 preparations per infant.[67,68] Surveys in Sweden and France have shown that 3 out of 4 infants between 6 months and 1 year of age receive commercially prepared baby foods.[69,70] They are generally not fortified with iron and there are no recommendations for their fortification. The average levels of iron in these products have been reported to be 0.21 mg/100 g for strained fruits and 0.51 mg/100 g for strained vegetables, 2.21 mg/100 g for strained meats, and 0.43 mg/100 g for vegetable and meat combination dinners.[66]

IV. IRON PREPARATIONS USED TO FORTIFY INFANT FOODS

The bioavailability of fortification iron depends on the effects of ligands in the meal that act on the common non-heme iron pool as well as the nature of the iron source itself. The interaction between food and non-heme iron has been discussed above and applies as much to fortification iron as it does to the native food iron. Factors affecting bioavailability that are dependent on the iron source itself include solubility in gastric juice and the facility with which it enters the common pool.[71,72]

In addition to bioavailability, considerations such as organoleptic properties and national regulations affect the choice of fortificants. Most countries have their own permitted lists. A Codex Alimentarius is also available.[73] Only the cost of the iron source is of minor importance. It adds less than 0.1% to the total price of the product.[71]

A. BIOAVAILABLITY OF FORTIFICATION IRON SOURCES

Since the absolute absorption of a given iron source is difficult to predict, food manufacturers use its relative bioavailability value (RBV) as a guide to its potential absorption. The RBV is obtained by measuring the absorption and utilization of a given iron source relative to ferrous sulfate (RBV for ferrous sulfate is set at 100). The RBV is usually measured in anemic rats using the hemoglobin repletion test.[74,75] Occasionally studies have been performed in iron-replete human volunteers with either pharmacological quantities of iron[76] or iron added to foods.[77] Iron sources with an RBV similar to ferrous sulfate are expected to be equally well utilized. The anticipated absorption of an equivalent amount of an iron source with a lower RBV would be correspondingly less; however, poorly soluble iron sources enter the common pool to a variable extent, and their relative bioavailability may not be predictable with certainty.[72]

In general, iron sources that are freely water soluble have a high relative bioavailability (Table 4). Those used in infant formulas, however, can usually not be used to fortify infant cereals because they affect both the color and the flavor.[78] Therefore, iron sources that are poorly soluble in water are usually added to infant cereals. Relative bioavailability is almost always low.

B. IRON SOURCES ADDED TO INFANT FORMULAS

Virtually all liquid and powdered infant formulas are fortified with ferrous sulfate in both the U.S. and Europe,[79] although other iron sources, such as ferrous gluconate,[80] ferrous lactate,[81,82] and ferrous ammonium citrate[83] have also been used. Each of these salts is on the permitted list in the Codex Alimentarius[73] and has been reported to have an RBV similar to ferrous sulfate. Ferrous citrate is also an approved iron salt, but is poorly soluble in water with an RBV of about 75 for both rats and human beings (Table 4).

C. IRON SOURCES ADDED TO INFANT CEREALS

Sodium iron pyrophosphate which was used commonly in the early 1970s is poorly bioavailable. It has been replaced by elemental iron which is widely used in the U.S. and ferric pyrophosphate, especially in Europe.

There are three types of elemental iron depending on the method of manufacture, reduced iron, electrolytic iron, and carbonyl iron.[84] Reduced iron is produced by exposing iron oxide powder to hydrogen or carbon monoxide. It consists of a sponge-like irregular porous particle. It usually has the largest mean particle size and has given the lowest RBV values for commercially available elemental iron sources.[85] Electrolytic iron is manufactured by the electrolytic deposition of iron from a ferrous sulfate bath onto thin stainless steel cathode sheets. It forms flat, irregular fern-like particles of high surface area. Carbonyl iron, which has been used mainly in Europe, is produced by heating scrap metal with pressurized carbon

TABLE 4
Relative Bioavailability of the Different Sources of Iron Used to Fortify Infant Foods

	Av. relative bioavailability[a]	
	Rat[b]	Human[c]
Sources added to infant formula		
Ferrous sulphate	100	100
Ferrous gluconate	97	89
Ferrous lactate	—	106
Ferric ammonium citrate	107	—
Ferrous citrate	76	74
Sources added to infant cereal		
Elemental iron	8—76	13—90
Ferric pyrophosphate	45	—
Ferric orthophosphate	7—32	31
Ferric saccharate	92	—
Ferrous fumarate	95	101
Ferrous succinate	119	123

[a] Measured relative to ferrous sulfate = 100.
[b] Hemoglobin repletion test; values from Fritz et al.[74] Fritz and Pla[75] and Hurrell.[71]
[c] Absorption measured using radioiron isotopes; values from Brise and Hallberg,[76] Cook et al.[77] and Björn-Rasmussen et al.[100]

monoxide to yield iron pentacarbonyl which is then decomposed to a powder. The particles are very small (0 to 10 μm) and spherical, often forming clusters. The RBV in rats has been reported to be about 60%, better than both reduced and the electrolytic iron.[85,86]

Due to variations in production, each type may itself vary in particle shape, size, and surface area. Bioavailablity depends on solubility in gastric juice and is governed as much by differences in particle size and surface area as the type of powder. Therefore, variation in bioavailability may be as great using the same type of product as when different products are compared.[78] In the earlier studies of electrolytically reduced iron, material of small particle size (5 to 10 μm) was used and bioavailability equal to that of ferrous sulfate was reported.[36] Unfortunately, these observations may not be representative of the electrolytic iron commonly used to fortify infant cereals in the U.S. which has a particle size ranging from 0 to 40 μm. Thus commercial electrolytic powders have given RBVs as low as 32 to 40.[78,85] Similar discrepancies between experimental and commercial products may apply to carbonyl iron. In a recent study of iron-replete healthy human subjects fed wheat rolls fortified with radioactively labeled carbonyl iron, Hallberg et al.[72] reported an RBV that varied from 5 to 33 depending on the type of meal in which the iron was eaten. The variation in the RBV appeared to be the result of different rates of dissolution of carbonyl iron in gastric juice as well as variation in the rate of gastric emptying. The unexpectedly low RBV of carbonyl iron led the workers to suggest that the use of elemental iron powders in fortification of human foods be reconsidered.

Ferric pyrophosphate has an RBV of 45 in the hemoglobin repletion test. Unfortunately, no reliable human studies have been performed. Its solubility may be improved by forming a coprecipitate with sodium citrate or ammonium citrate. These double salts have RBVs similar to ferrous sulfate, but may cause organoleptic problems when added to infant cereals.[71] Ferric orthophosphate and ferric saccharate are occasionally added to infant cereals by European companies. Ferric orthophosphate has a low and variable RBV while ferric saccharate is well utilized, but its brown color may cause discoloration when higher levels are added.

Ferrous succinate and ferrous fumarate are the best alternatives to elemental iron and ferric pyrophosphate for infant cereal fortification. Organoleptic problems have not been encountered at fortification levels up to 50 mg iron per 100 g food.[102] In rat and human studies, the RBV has been similar to or better than that of ferrous sulfate. Although both are insoluble in water, they dissolve readily in dilute acids. Both are on the Codex permitted list for infant foods. Ferrous fumarate is already in use in the U.S. About 3% of infant cereals are fortified with this form of iron.[79]

D. INFLUENCE OF PROCESSING ON BIOAVAILABILITY OF IRON SOURCES

Heat sterilization of infant formula increases the relative bioavailability of poorly bioavailable iron sources, such as ferric pyrophosphate and sodium iron pyrophosphate, and has little effect on available iron salts, such as ferrous sulfate.[81,82] On the other hand, the processing of poorly available iron salts in cereal products, such as bread rolls[77] or mixed infant cereal[87] does not appear to improve iron bioavailability.

V. METHODS FOR IMPROVING BIOAVAILABILITY OF IRON IN INFANT FOODS

The fortification of food with sufficient iron to supply the infant's needs despite poor bioavailability is the strategy for preventing iron deficiency in young children that has been adopted almost universally; however, some foods are very inhibitory, necessitating the addition of large amounts of iron. An alternative approach is the use of measures to improve bioavailability. Three methods have been examined experimentally. They are the addition of an enhancer of iron absorption to the food, the use of a form of iron that does not enter the non-heme common pool and is yet available for absorption, and the processing of food items to modify their inhibitory properties.

A. ENHANCERS OF IRON ABSORPTION

The addition of ascorbic acid to improve iron bioavailability has been studied by several investigators[88] and appears to be the most practical approach. In one study, measurements of iron bioavailability from an instant milk formula and three infant cereals demonstrated that absorption was increased significantly when ascorbic acid was added.[89] The effect was dose dependent and similar for the three fortification sources tested, ferrous sulfate, ferric pyrophosphate, and ferric ammonium citrate. Two recent publications provide additional precise, quantitative information on the effect of ascorbic acid in infant formulas. In one, absorption was measured in adults,[90] while in the other 5- to 18-month-old infants were studied.[91] The results are remarkably similar and demonstrate that ascorbic acid improves the absorption of iron from milk formulas in a dose-dependent fashion until a maximum effect is obtained at about a 4:1 molar ratio of ascorbic acid to iron (usually about 200 mg ascorbic acid per liter formula). A similar proportional effect was obtained using a soy-based formula, but absorption in the absence of ascorbic acid was so low that the improvement in absolute absorption was relatively small.[90] The quantity of iron absorbed still fell short of a 1-year-old infant's requirements.

While infant formulas and other baby foods are usually fortified with vitamin C to ensure an adequate supply of this essential nutrient, no attempt has been made to use vitamin C fortification as a systematic means for improving iron nutrition in infancy; however, a preliminary field trial conducted in Chile demonstrated the potential benefit of this approach.[92] The International Nutritional Anemia Consultative Group (INACG) have also recently recommended the addition of an adequate quantity of ascorbic acid to cereal-soy blended foods to enhance bioavailability.[37] It should be noted that the benefit of ascorbic acid may be lost because of oxidation during storage or prolonged warming of meals.[93] however, the use of cellulose-coated ascorbic acid may reduce degradation with very little increase in cost.[94]

The chelate ethylene diamine tetraacetic acid (EDTA) also appears to have an overriding effect on the common non-heme iron pool, but its properties are different from those of ascorbic acid. It forms a stable complex with the iron in the pool which appears to be protected to some extent from inhibiting ligands. As with ascorbic acid, the molar ratio of EDTA to iron becomes the determinant of percentage iron absorption, but in contradistinction to the former compound a significant inhibitory effect is observed in meals containing molar ratios above 2:1. When Fe EDTA is prepared by mixing equimolar solutions of disodium EDTA and ferric chloride, and added to maize, porridge, or bran, however, iron absorption is adequate and relatively little affected by the inhibitory factors present, whereas the absorption of ferrous sulfate is markedly reduced.[95-98] On the other hand, the enhancing effect of ascorbic acid is much less pronounced with Fe (III) EDTA than it is with ferrous sulfate.[96]

These studies show that sodium iron EDTA is attractive as a potential form of iron for fortification because, its absorption is relatively predictable and less markedly affected by meal composition than are other iron sources. It has been used extensively as a food fortificant in government and university programs, having been added to sugar, milk, fish sauce, curry powder, and various cereals. These studies have been reviewed in detail recently.[98]

Sodium iron EDTA is not on the Codex permitted list, but sodium calcium EDTA is widely used as a food preservative in the U.S. Unfortunately, EDTA is absorbed and then excreted in the urine. There are thus theoretical concerns that its long-term use could interfere with the metabolism of calcium and other minerals. It seems unlikely that this compound will be used to fortify infant foods in the near future.

B. ISOLATION FOR FORTIFICATION IRON FROM THE NONHEME COMMON POOL

Iron bioavailability could be improved by protecting a potentially well-absorbed form of iron from the common pool ligands. Two experimental approaches are feasible. Encapsulated ferrous sulfate has been made by using hydrogenated oils, maltodextrin, zinc stearate, and ethyl cellulose. The capsule prevents fat oxidation reactions and the occurrence of flavor changes. Moreover, with the possible exception of zinc stearate capsules, there is little or no reduction in the absorption and utilization of the iron in the anemic rats.[71] Unfortunately, the capsule may be destroyed by food preparation leading to discoloration of foods, such as infant cereals before consumption.[78]

A second approach would take advantage of the consistently high bioavailability of iron in the heme pool which is not affected by the inhibitory ligands operating in the non-heme pool. Spray-dried bovine blood has been used to fortify cookies provided to children as a part of a school lunch program in Chile. Each 30-g cookie contained 5 mg hemoglobin iron, 20% of which was absorbed.[98] The major drawback of this method of fortification lies in the low iron content of hemoglobin (0.31%) as well as its color. It would be necessary to add 3.2 g of hemoglobin to an infant cereal to provide 10 mg iron, leading to unacceptable changes in color. Moreover, it might be difficult to guarantee a regular supply of pathogen-free blood and provide for appropriate storage.

C. MODIFICATION OF INHIBITORY FACTORS IN BABY FOODS

The most direct method of improving iron availability is the removal or modification of the inhibitory factors themselves. This approach has received least attention, probably because of the widely held belief that numerous different inhibitors play a role in any particular food. Our ignorance of the precise nature of these ligands makes attempts to reduce their effects difficult. One simple approach to modifying inhibitory ligands, that of heating, has been tested experimentally with soybeans and egg white.[99] In both instances a modest improvement in bioavailability was achieved. Unfortunately, it does not represent a practical approach at the present time because of unacceptable changes in the functional properties of the food and potential damage to other nutrients; however, other methods may merit further study. In this context, our recent observations demonstrating that the inhibitory properties of several purified proteins can be virtually removed by partial hydrolysis of the protein are of some interest.[27]

ACKNOWLEDGMENT

This work was supported by AID Cooperative Agreement DAN-0227-A-00-2104-00.

REFERENCES

1. **Dallman, P. R., Siimes, M. A., and Stekel, A.,** Iron deficiency in infancy and childhood, *Am. J. Clin. Nutr.,* 33, 86, 1980.
2. **Smith, N. J. and Rios, E.,** Iron metabolism and iron deficiency in infancy and childhood, *Adv. Pediatr.,* 21, 239, 1974.
3. **Stekel, A.,** Iron requirements in infancy and childhood, in *Iron Nutrition in Infancy and Childhood,* Stekel, A., Ed., Nestlé, Vevey/Raven Press, New York, 1984, 1.
4. **Elian, E., Bar-Shani, S., Liberman, A., and Matoth, Y.,** Intestinal blood loss: a factor in calculations of body iron in late infancy, *J. Pediatr.,* 69, 215, 1966.
5. **Rasch, C. A., Cotton, E. K., Harris, J. W., and Griggs, R. C.,** Blood loss as a contributing factor in the etiology of iron-lack anemia of infancy, *Am. J. Dis. Child.,* 100, 627, 1960.
6. **Hoag, M. S., Wallerstein, R. O., and Pollycove, M.,** Occult blood loss in iron deficiency anemia of infancy, *Pediatrics,* 27, 199, 1961.
7. **Wilson, J. F., Heiner, D. C., and Lahey, M. E.,** Milk-induced gastrointestinal bleeding in infants with hypochromic-microcytic anemia, *JAMA,* 189, 568, 1964.
8. **Woodruff, C. W., Wright, S. W., and Wright, R. P.,** The role of fresh cow's milk in iron deficiency. II. Comparison of fresh cow's milk with a prepared formula, *Am. J. Dis. Child.,* 124, 26, 1972.
9. **Wilson, J. F., Lahey, M. E., and Heiner, D. C.,** Studies on iron metabolism. V. Further observations on cow's milk-induced gastrointestinal bleeding in infants with iron-deficiency anemia, *J. Pediatr.,* 84, 335, 1974.
10. **Siimes, M. A., Salmenperä, L., and Perheentupa, J.,** Exclusive breast-feeding for 9 months: risk of iron deficiency, *J. Pediatr.,* 104, 196, 1984.
11. **Lönnerdal, B.,** Iron and breast milk, in *Iron Nutrition in Infancy and Childhood,* Stekel, A., Ed., Nestlé, Vevey/Raven Press, New York, 1984, 95.
12. **McMillan, J. A., Landaw, S. A., and Oski, F.,** Iron sufficiency in breast-fed infants and the availability of iron from human milk, *Pediatrics,* 58, 686, 1976.
13. **Bothwell, T. H., Charlton, R. W., Cook, J. D., and Finch, C. A.,** *Iron Metabolism in Man,* Blackwell Scientific, Oxford, 1979.
14. **Björn-Rasmussen, E., Hallberg, L., Isaksson, B., and Arvidsson, B.,** Food iron absorption in man. Applications of the two-pool extrinsic tag method to measure heme and nonheme iron absorption from the whole diet, *J. Clin. Invest.,* 53, 247, 1974.
15. American Academy of Pediatrics, Committee on Nutrition, Iron supplementation for infants, *Pediatrics,* 58, 765, 1976.
16. **Cook, J. D., Layrisse, M., and Finch, C. A.,** The measurement of iron absorption, *Blood,* 33, 421, 1969.
17. **Moore, C. V. and Dubach, R.,** Observations on the absorption of iron from foods tagged with radioiron, *Trans. Assoc. Am. Phys.,* 64, 245, 1951.
18. **Cook, J. D., Layrisse, M., Martinez-Torres, C., Walker, R., Monsen, E., and Finch, C. A.,** Food iron absorption measured by an extrinsic tag, *J. Clin. Invest.,* 51, 805, 1972.
19. **Björn-Rasmussen, E., Hallberg, L., and Walker R. B.,** Food iron absorption in man. 1. Isotopic exchange between food iron and inorganic iron salts added to food: studies on maize, wheat and eggs, *Am. J. Clin. Nutr.,* 25, 317, 1972.

20. **Hallberg, L., Björn-Rasmussen, E., Garby, L., Pleehachinda, R., and Suwanik, R.,** Iron absorption from South-East Asian diets and the effect of iron fortification, *Am. J. Clin. Nutr.,* 31, 1403, 1978.
21. **Layrisse, M., Martinez-Torres, C., Renzi, M., and Leets, I.,** Ferritin iron absorption in man, *Blood,* 45, 689, 1975.
22. **Derman, D., Sayers, M., Lynch, S. R., Charlton, R. W., Bothwell, T. H., and Mayet, F.,** Iron absorption from a cereal-based meal containing cane sugar fortified with ascorbic acid, *Br. J. Nutr.,* 38, 261, 1977.
23. **Hallberg, L. and Björn-Rasmussen, E.,** Measurement of iron absorption from meals contaminated with iron, *Am. J. Clin. Nutr.,* 34, 2808, 1981.
24. **Magnusson, B., Björn-Rasmussen, E., Rossander, L., and Hallberg, L.,** Iron absorption in relation to iron status. Model proposed to express results of food iron absorption measurements, *Scand. J. Haematol.,* 27, 201, 1981.
25. **Ashworth, A. and March Y.,** Iron fortification of dried skim milk and maize-soya-bean-milk mixture (CSM): availability of iron in Jamaican infants, *Br. J. Nutr.,* 30, 577, 1973.
26. **McMillan, J. A., Oski, F. A., Lourie, G., Tomarelli, R. M., and Landaw, S. A.,** Iron absorption from human milk, simulated human milk, and proprietary formulas, *Pediatrics,* 60, 896, 1977.
27. **Lynch, S. R., Hurrell, R., Dassenko, S. A., and Cook, J. D.,** The effect of protein on nonheme iron bioavailability, *Clin. Res.,* 34, 800A, 1986.
28. **Miller, D. D., Schricker, B. R., Rasmussen, R. R., and Van Campen, D.,** An *in vitro* method for estimation of iron availability from meals, *Am. J. Clin. Nutr.,* 34, 2248, 1981.
29. **Cook, J. D. and Bothwell, T. H.,** Availability of iron from infant foods, in *Iron Nutrition in Infancy and Childhood,* Stekel A., Ed., Nestlé, Vevey/Raven Press, New York, 1984, 119.
30. **Cook, J. D. and Monsen, E. R.,** Food iron absorption III Comparison of the effect of animal proteins on non-heme iron absorption, *Am. J. Clin. Nutr.,* 29, 859, 1976.
31. **Layrisse, M., Cook, J. D., Martinez-Torres, C., Roche, M., Kuhn, I. N., Walker, R. B., and Finch, C. A.,** Food iron absorption: a comparison of vegetable and animal foods, *Blood,* 33, 430, 1969.
32. **Sayers, M. H., Lynch, S. R., Jacobs, P., Charlton, R. W., Bothwell, T. H., Walker, R. B., and Mayet, F.,** The effects of ascorbic acid supplementation on the absorption of iron in maize, wheat and soya, *Br. J. Haematol.,* 24, 209, 1973.
33. **Björn-Rasmussen, E., Hallberg, L., and Walker, R. B.,** Food iron absorption in man. II. Isotopic exchange of iron between labelled foods and between a food and an iron salt, *Am. J. Clin. Nutr.,* 26, 1311, 1973.
34. **Cook, J. D., Morck, T. A., and Lynch, S. R.,** The inhibitory effect of soy products on nonheme iron absorption in man, *Am. J. Clin. Nutr.,* 34, 2622, 1981.
35. **Morck, T. A., Lynch, S. R., Skikne, B. S., and Cook, J. D.,** Iron availability from infant food supplements, *Am. J. Clin. Nutr.,* 34, 2630, 1981.
36. **Rios, E., Hunter, R. E., Cook, J. D., Smith, N. J., and Finch, C. A.,** The absorption of iron as supplements in infant cereal and infant formulas, *Pediatrics,* 55, 686, 1975.
37. International Nutritional Anemia Consultative Group, *Iron Absorption from Cereals and Legumes. A Report of the Nutritional Anemia Consultative Group,* The Nutrition Foundation, New York, 1982.
38. **Lynch, S. R., Beard, J. L., Dassenko, S. A., and Cook, J. D.,** Iron absorption from legumes in humans, *Am. J. Clin. Nutr.,* 40, 42, 1984.
39. **Disler, P. B., Lynch, S. R., Charlton R. W., Torrance, J. D., Bothwell, T. H., Walker R. B., and Mayet F.,** The effect of tea on iron absorption, *Gut,* 16, 193, 1975.
40. **Reddy, N. R., Sathe, S. K., and Salunkhe, D. K.,** Phytates in legumes and cereals, *Adv. Food Res.,* 28, 1, 1982.
41. **Beard, J., Weaver, C. M., Lynch, S., Johnson, C. O., Dassenko, S. A., and Cook, J. D.,** The effect of soybean phytate content on iron bioavailability, in preparation.
42. **Björn-Rasmussen, E.,** Iron absorption from wheat bread. Influence of various amounts of bran, *Nutr. Metab.,* 16, 101, 1974.
43. **Simpson, K. M., Morris, E. R., and Cook, J. D.,** The inhibitory effect of bran on iron absorption in man, *Am. J. Clin. Nutr.,* 34, 1469, 1981.
44. **Lipschitz, D. A., Simpson, K. M., Cook, J. D., and Morris, E. R.,** Absorption of monoferric phytate by dogs, *J. Nutr.,* 109, 1154, 1979.
45. Committee on Dietary Allowances, Food and Nutritional Board, National Research Council, *Recommended Dietary Allowances,* 9th ed., National Academy of Sciences, Washington, D.C., 1980.
46. **Montalto, M. B., Benson, J. D., and Martinez, G. A.,** Nutrient intakes of formula-fed infants and infants fed cow's milk, *Pediatrics,* 75, 343, 1985.
47. American Academy of Pediatrics, Committee on Nutrition, The use of whole cow's milk in infancy, *Pediatrics,* 72, 253, 1983.
48. **Gurr, M. I.,** Review of the progress of dairy science: human and artificial milks for infant feeding, *J. Dairy Res.,* 48, 519, 1981.

49. ESPGAN Committee on Nutrition, Guidelines on infant nutrition, I. Recommendations for the composition of an adapted formula, *Acta. Paediatr. Scand.*, Suppl. 262, 1977.
50. ESPGAN Committee on Nutrition, Guidelines on infant nutrition, II. Recommendations for the composition of follow-up formula and beikost, *Acta. Paediatr. Scand.*, Suppl. 287, 1, 1981.
51. Codex, Alimentarius Commission, Codex Standards for Foods for Special Dietary Uses Including Foods for Infants and Young Children and Related Code of Hygienic Practice, CAL/VOL IX, Joint FAO/WHO food standards programme, FAO, Rome, 1982.
52. **DuBois, I. M.,** Legislation on infant formula and its impact on food manufacturers, in *Production, Regulation and Analysis of Infant Formula*, Association of Official Analytical Chemists, Arlington, VA, 1985, 38.
53. **Woodruff, C. W.,** American Academy of Pediatrics, Committee on Nutrition, Perspectives on Infant Formula, in *Production, Regulation and Analysis of Infant Formula*, Association of Official Analytical Chemists, Arlington, VA, 1985, 15.
54. American Academy of Pediatrics, Committee on Nutrition, Commentary on breast-feeding and infant formulas, including proposed standards for formulas, *Pediatrics*, 57, 278, 1976.
55. **Weinberg, E. D.,** Iron and susceptiblity to infectious disease, *Science*, 184, 952, 1974.
56. American Academy of Pediatrics, Committee on Nutrition, Relationship between iron status and incidence of infection in infancy, *Pediatrics*, 62, 246, 1978.
57. **Oski, F. A.,** Iron-fortified formulas and gastrointestinal symptoms in infants: a controlled study, *Pediatrics*, 66, 168, 1980.
58. **Widdowson, E. M., Southgate, D. A. T., and Schutz, Y.,** Comparison of dried milk preparations for babies on sale in 7 European countries I. Protein, fat, carbohydrate and inorganic constituents, *Arch. Dis. Child.*, 49, 867, 1974.
59. **Kirkpatrick, D. C., Conacher, H. B. S., Méranger, J. C., Dabeka, R., Collins, B., McKenzie, A. D., Lacroix, G. M. A., and Savary, G.,** The trace element content of Canadian baby foods and estimation of trace element intake by infants, *Can. Inst. Food Sci. Technol. J.*, 13, 154, 1980.
60. **Muzzarelli, R. A. A., Eugeni, C. E., Tanfani, F., Caramia, G., and Pezzola, D.,** Atomic absorption determination of chromium, manganese, iron, copper, and zinc in human, cow's and powdered milks, *Milchwissenschaft*, 38, 453, 1983.
61. **Lönnerdal, B., Keen, C. L., Ohtake, M., and Tamura, T.,** Iron, zinc, copper and manganese in infant formulas, *Am. J. Dis. Child.*, 137, 433, 1983.
62. **Kelly, V. J.,** The use of cereal grains in infant feeding, *Cereal Foods World*, 29, 721, 1984.
63. U.S. Food and Drug Administration Rules and Regulations (Part 125), Label Statements Concerning Dietary Properties of Food Purporting to be of Represented for Special Dietary Uses. *Fed. Regist.*, 36(238), 23, 553, 1971.
64. **Yeung, D. L., Pennell, M. D., Leung, M., Hall, J., and Anderson, G. H.,** Iron intake in infants: the importance of infant cereals, *Can. Med. Assoc. J.*, 125, 999, 1981.
65. Societé Francaise de Pédiatrie, Comité de Nutrition, Le fer dans l'alimentation du nourisson, *Arch. Fr. Pediatr.*, 37, 337, 1980.
66. **Deeming, S. B. and Weber, C. W.,** Trace minerals in commercially prepared baby foods, *J. Am. Diet. Assoc.*, 75, 149, 1979.
67. **Fomon, S. J.,** *Infant Nutrition*, 2nd ed., W. B. Sanders, Philadelphia, 1974.
68. **Astier-Dumas, M.,** Les aliments de l'enfance, farines de céreales et préparations spéciales en petits pots. Le point de vue du nutritioniste, *Rev. Pediatr.*, 11, 229, 1975.
69. **Kohler, E. M., Kohler, L., and Lindquist, B.,** Use of weaning foods (Beikost) in an industrialized society. Socio-economic and physiological aspects, *Acta Paediatr. Scand.*, 66, 665, 1977.
70. **Lestradet, H., Machinot, S., Greneche, M. O., Dufur, C., and Six, M. F.,** L'alimentation des nourrissons francais de 2 a 9 mois. Etude qualitative et quantitative, *Rev. Pediatr.*, 15, 11, 1979.
71. **Hurrell, R. F.,** II. Types of iron fortificants, Nonelemental Sources, in *Iron Fortification of Foods*, Clydesdale, F. M. and Wiemer, K. L., Eds., Academic Press, Orlando, FL, 1985, 39.
72. **Hallberg, L., Brune, M., and Rossander, L.,** Low bioavailablity of carbonyl iron in man: studies on iron fortification of wheat flour, *Am. J. Clin. Nutr.*, 43, 59, 1986.
73. Codex Alimentarius Commission, *Report of Codex Committee on Foods for Special Dietary Uses*, Alinorm 81/26, Joint FAO/WHO Food Standards Programme, Food and Agriculture Organization, Rome, 1981.
74. **Fritz, J. C., Pla, G. W., Roberts, T., Boehne, J. W., and Hove, E. L.,** Biological availability in animals of iron from common dietary sources, *J. Agric. Food Chem.*, 18, 647, 1970.
75. **Fritz, J. C. and Pla, G. W.,** Application of the animal hemoglobin repletion test to measurement of iron availability in foods, *J. Assoc. Off. Anal. Chem.*, 55, 1128, 1972.
76. **Brise, H. and Hallberg, L.,** A method for comparative studies on iron absorption in man using two radioiron isotopes, *Acta Med. Scand.*, 171(Suppl. 376), 7, 1962.
77. **Cook, J. D., Minnich, V., Moore, C. V., Rasmussen, A., Bradley, W. B., and Finch, C. A.,** Absorption of fortification iron in bread, *Am. J. Clin. Nutr.*, 26, 861, 1973.

78. **Hurrell, R. F.,** Bioavailability of different iron compounds used to fortify formulas and cereals: technological problems, in *Iron Nutrition in Infancy and Childhood,* Stekel, A., Ed., Nestlé, Vevey/Raven Press, New York, 1984, 147.

79. **Rees, J. M., Monsen, E. R., and Merrill, J. E.,** Iron fortification of infant foods. A decade of change, *Clin. Pediatr.,* 24, 707, 1985.

80. **Saarinen, U. M. and Siimes, M. A.** Iron absorption from breast milk, cow's milk and iron-supplemented formula: an opportunistic use of changes in total body iron determined by haemoglobin, ferritin and body weight in 132 infants, *Pediatr. Res.,* 13, 143, 1979.

81. **Theuer, R. C., Kemmerer, K. S., Martin, W. H., Zoumas, B. L., and Sarett, H. P.,** Effect of processing on availability of iron salts in liquid infant formula products: experimental soy isolate formulas, *J. Agric. Food Chem.,* 19, 555, 1971.

82. **Theuer, R. C., Martin, W. H., Wallander, J. F., and Sarett, H. P.,** Effect of processing on availability of iron salts in liquid infant formula products: experimental milk-based formulas, *J. Agric. Food Chem.,* 21, 482, 1973.

83. **Cook, J. D. and Reusser, M. E.,** Iron fortification: an update, *Am. J. Clin. Nutr.,* 38, 648, 1983.

84. **Patrick, J.,** Types of iron fortificants. Elemental sources, in *Iron Fortification of Foods,* Clydesdale, F. M. and Wiemer, K. L., Eds., Academic Press, Orlando, FL, 1985, 31.

85. **Shah, B. G., Giroux, A., and Belonje, B.,** Specifications for reduced iron as a food additive, *J. Agric. Food Chem.,* 27, 845, 1977.

86. **Fritz, J. C.,** Bioavailability of mineral nutrients, *Chemtech,* 6, 643, 1976.

87. **Rees, J. M. and Monsen, E. R.,** Absorption of fortification iron by the rat: comparison of type and level of iron incorporation into mixed grain cereal, *J. Agric. Food Chem.,* 21, 913, 1973.

88. **Lynch, S. R. and Cook J. D.** Interaction of Vitamin C and iron, *Ann. N.Y. Acad. Sci.,* 355, 32, 1980.

89. **Derman, D. P., Bothwell, T. H., MacPhail, A. P., Torrance, J. D., Bezwoda, W. R., Charlton, R. W., and Mayet, F. G. H.,** Importance of ascorbic acid in the absorption of iron from infant foods, *Scand. J. Haematol.,* 25, 193, 1980.

90. **Gillooly, M., Torrance, J. D., Bothwell, T. H., MacPhail, A. P., Derman, D., Mills, W., and Mayet, F.,** The relative effect of ascorbic acid on iron absorption from soy-based and milk-based infant formulas, *Am. J. Clin. Nutr.,* 40, 522, 1984.

91. **Stekel, A., Olivares, M., Pizarro, F., Chadud, P., Lopez, I., and Amar, M.,** Absorption of fortification iron from milk formulas in infants, *Am. J. Clin. Nutr.,* 43, 917, 1986.

92. **Stekel, A., Olivares, M., Lopez, I., Amar, M., Pizarro, F., Chadud, P., Llaguno, S., and Cayazzo, M.,** Prevention of iron deficiency in infants by milk fortification, in *Nutrition Intervention Strategies in National Development,* Underwood, B. A., Ed., Academic Press, New York, 1983, 315.

93. **Hallberg, L., Rossander, L., Persson, H., and Svahn, E.,** Deleterious effects of prolonged warming of meals on ascorbic acid content and iron absorption, *Am. J. Clin. Nutr.,* 36, 846, 1982.

94. **Bookwalter, G. N., Bothast, R. J., Kwolek, W. F., and Gumbmann, M. R.,** Nutritional stability of corn-soy-milk blends after dry heating to destroy Salmonellae, *J. Food Sci.,* 45, 975, 1980.

95. **Viteri, F. E., Garcia-Ibanez, R., and Torun, B.,** Sodium iron NaFeEDTA as an iron fortification compound in Central America. Absorption Studies, *Am. J. Clin. Nutr.,* 31, 961, 1978.

96. **MacPhail, A. P., Bothwell, T. H., Torrance, J. D., Derman, D. P., Bezwoda, W. R., Charlton, R. W., and Mayet, F.,** Factors affecting the absorption of iron from Fe(111)EDTA, *Br. J. Nutr.,* 45, 215, 1981.

97. **Candela, E., Camacho, M. V., Martínez-Torres, C., Perdomo, J., Mazzarri, G., Acurero, G., and Layrisse, M.,** Iron absorption by human and swine from Fe(111)-EDTA. Further studies, *J. Nutr.,* 114, 2204, 1984.

98. **McPhail, P., Charlton, R., Bothwell, T. H., and Bezwoda, W.,** II. Types of iron fortificants. Experimental fortificants, in *Iron Fortification of Foods,* Clydesdale, F. M. and Wiemer, K. L., Eds., Academic Press, Orlando, FL, 1985, 55.

99. **Morck, T. A., Lynch, S. R., and Cook, J. D.,** Reduction of the soy-induced inhibition of nonheme iron absorption, *Am. J. Clin. Nutr.,* 36, 219, 1982.

100. **Björn-Rasmussen, E., Hallberg, L., and Rossander, L.,** Absorption of 'fortification' iron. Bioavailability in man of different samples of reduced Fe, and prediction of the effects of Fe fortification, *Br. J. Nutr.,* 37, 375, 1977.

101. **Cook, J. D., Lynch, S. R., and Skikne, B. S.,** unpublished observations.

102. **Burri, J. and Hurrell, R. F.,** unpublished observations.

Chapter 7

FIELD TRIALS OF FOOD FORTIFICATION WITH IRON: THE EXPERIENCE IN CHILE

Tomás Walter, Manuel Olivares, and Eva Hertrampf

TABLE OF CONTENTS

I. INTRODUCTION

Iron deficiency is one of the most common nutritional disorders. It is prevalent in most of the developing world and it is probably the only nutritional deficiency of consideration in industrialized countries. For physiologic reasons seen in previous chapters, the most commonly affected groups are infants, preschool children, adolescents, and women of child-bearing age. In the underdeveloped world, the prevalence is usually greatest in infants and to a lesser extent in women; in contrast, in industrialized countries, it is present mainly in women due to the additional iron requirements imposed by menstruation and pregnancy.

The only way that nutritional iron deficiency can be alleviated is by increasing iron intake either by providing medicinal iron (supplementation) or by adding iron to the diet (fortification). Iron supplementation can be directed to those populations at greatest risk and has the advantage of producing rapid changes in iron status. However, its effectiveness is limited because of the difficulty in sustaining the motivation of the participants, who may be additionally discouraged by the common occurrence of gastrointestinal side effects. Moreover, supplementation requires an effective system of health care delivery and is relatively costly to maintain. It is the most widely used way to prevent iron deficiency during pregnancy, when a relatively short period of time is required, individuals are easily recognizable, motivated, and usually accessible to the health care providers. On the other hand, the enormous increase in iron requirements imposed by pregnancy, cannot be met by the usual diet alone. Fortification is generally accepted as the best all around approach for combatting iron deficiency. It can be made to reach all sectors of the population, does not require the cooperation of the individual, the initial cost is small, and the maintenance expense is less than that of supplementation. However, there are technical difficulties in fortifying the diet with iron, many of which are discussed below.

While the selection of the food vehicle and fortificant iron source are considerations of importance, they have been recently reviewed,[1] and we address only those aspects relevant to our experience. There are other views, however, on the development of a fortification program that we attempt to outline. Prevalence studies are needed at the onset to establish that iron deficiency is sufficiently widespread to warrant a national intervention program. Having already determined the need for fortification, dietary surveys are indispensable to characterize the original diets with respect to their content of heme and non-heme iron as well as factors that may enhance or inhibit iron absorption. It is important to measure the actual iron absorption from the original diets in human subjects. This is usually accomplished using the extrinsic radioiron method. These dietary surveys and absorption studies are needed for determining whether the major problem is of limited iron intake, low bioavailability, or a combination of both and for estimating the level of iron fortification that will eventually be required to reduce the prevalence of iron deficiency. This exercise has been recently performed for typical Latin American diets.[2]

An illustration of the previous point can be taken from the experience in Sweden described by Hallberg[3] where over a period of 40 years, the level of iron fortification in white wheat flour was increased from 3 mg to 6.5 mg of iron per 100 g of flour. The prevalence of iron deficiency anemia in Swedish women also decreased from 25 to 30% to 5 to 10%. However, this fall in incidence of anemia cannot readily be attributed only to fortification since other factors that affect iron stores had also taken effect, such as changes in contraceptive techniques and dietary habits. Consequently, to quantify the contribution of wheat fortification detailed knowledge is needed regarding (1) iron requirements, (2) iron absorption from the diet, and (3) bioavailability of fortification iron. Knowing the amount of fortificant that reached the target group, the relative bioavailability of the iron compound and the bioavailability of the non-heme iron in the meal containing the fortification iron, it was then necessary to know the prevalence of iron deficiency in this group and the distribution of

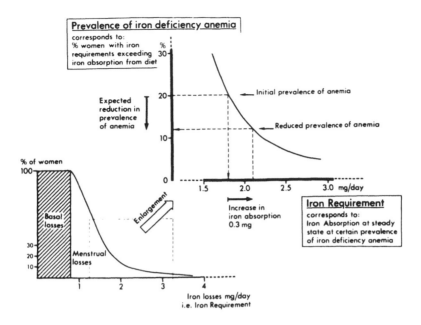

FIGURE 1. Iron requirements of Swedish women. The figure at the left depicts iron losses of women in fertile age. The enlargement at the right shows that an increase in absorption in 0.2 mg iron per day will reduce the prevalence of anemia in 8%. That is to say, it will offset the losses in excess of 1.8 mg/d to slightly above 2 mg/d. (From Hallberg, L., *Semin. Hematol.*, 19, 31, 1982. With permission.)

iron requirements in the population at large. The rationale for such a calculation has been published in detail,[3] but a simplified outline is illustrated in Figure 1. The cumulative distribution of iron requirements in menstruating women is shown in this figure where the ordinate represents the percent of women with different iron losses and shows that 20% of them sustain a daily iron loss in excess of 1.8 mg. If the prevalence of iron deficiency is 20%, then this relationship implies that the diet can offset a daily iron loss of at least 1.8 mg/d. If iron fortification is calculated to give a total absorption increase of 0.3 mg in the borderline subjects, then the prevalence of iron deficiency will fall to 12%. If instead, the initial prevalence were only 10%, then the effect of the same absorption increase would be a smaller reduction in prevalence reflecting a difference in the slope of the distribution curve of the iron requirement of these women. These calculations however, are only applicable for the Swedish diet and it is now well known that dietary factors profoundly affect the bioavailability of iron in the diet. Every country and even every region must estimate the dietary iron present and its bioavailability from the typical diet. Since these diets are very variable, it is appealing to introduce the concept of "bioavailable nutrient density iron", that is, the amount of iron bioavailable for 1000 kcal of intake.[4] If the bioavailable nutrient density is known and the average caloric intake is also known, the amount of iron that must be added to the diet (and its bioavailability) can be estimated for the prevention of iron deficiency in most of the population. In Figure 2, the bioavailable nutrient density of iron has been calculated for Swedish diets and the bioavailable iron is depicted for the different levels of energy intake of the population. These estimates need to be taken into account when calculating the biavailable nutrient density for diets of infants, women, and other population groups.

After all these appraisals have been completed and the selection of fortificant and the vehicle have been adequately studied, the most costly and time-consuming step before the development of a National Fortification Policy is conducting a field trial to establish its efficacy. The steps to consider in delineating a fortification policy are outlined in Table 1.

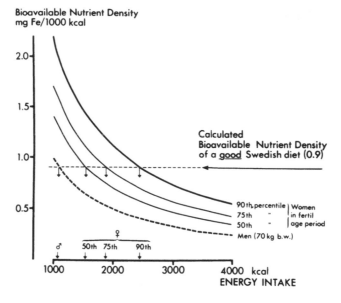

FIGURE 2.   Bioavailable iron nutrient density needed at different energy intakes to cover iron requirements in men and a certain portion of menstruating women. The dotted horizontal line is the estimated bioavailable nutrient density (0.9 mg/1000 kcal) of a good Swedish diet today. (From Hallberg, L., *Semin. Hematol.*, 19, 31, 1982. With permission.)

TABLE 1
Steps in Planning a Regional Fortification Program

Evaluate prevalence of iron deficiency
— Select target groups
— Study diets and dietary habits
— Study dietary content of heme and non-heme iron
— Study the absorption of dietary iron in typical diets
— Select vehicle and iron fortificant
— Select the level of fortification necessary
— Evaluate absorption enhancers, if necessary
— Study absorption of iron from fortified food
— Study acceptability of fortified food in the laboratory
— Field trial to study biologic effect and acceptability
— Field trial to study biologic effect, acceptability,
  and feasibility in the original conditions of the product
  distribution and consumption
— Plan future evaluation of impact

The field trial ought to be designed in order to evaluate several issues. The acceptability of the vehicle is established by laboratory methodology, i.e., the organoleptic qualities of the food products tested by a panel of judges. Then, acceptability and biological effectiveness trials are conducted in a pilot field study of a few hundred individuals. The actual number will depend on the expected changes in hematological measurements in order to attain statistically valid conclusions. At a second stage, the field trial needs to be planned to test the product's attributes, utilizing the health infrastructure and the food delivery systems that normally operate for consumption of the foods to be fortified. This is a crucial step to ensure the efficacy as well as the durability of the program since fortification of food products is intended as a long-term approach to the eradication of iron deficiency. After the effectiveness of the planned fortification has been tested in the pilot field situation and the expanded field situation just referred to, provisions should be made to permit the long-term evaluation of this program. Regions could either be left unfortified or preferably evaluated prospectively at periodic intervals.

In the evaluation of the field trial, several aspects need to be carefully controlled as mentioned previously. Field studies may fail to demonstrate the beneficial effect of fortification for a variety of reasons. The fortification level may be too low, the bioavailability of fortification iron may be insufficient because of unforeseen inhibitory effects of the usual diet, poor consumer acceptance, or error in the laboratory assessment of the iron status of the population. The duration of the trial may be too short to assure a statistically significant effect, particularly in the case of populations with only a low or moderate prevalence of iron deficiency. The study may have been designed in a suboptimal fashion so as to prevent adequate statistical evaluation. Investigation of other factors that may influence the reliability of results must be implemented, such as measurement of quantities of fortified products consumed (by dietary surveys) or by other means, such as the measurement of stool iron (a useful method in infants). Morbidity data, particularly for gastrointestinal disorders is important, when they are common in the target community, since it may influence iron absorption or increase iron losses, or may be inadvertently related to the fortified food. It is also possible that the community attributes the illness (diarrhea or constipation) to the introduction of the fortified food, thus limiting its acceptability. Finally, the anemia under investigation could be due to causes other than iron deficiency. In the following chapter, we attempt to illustrate many of these issues as they have been presented during our experience.

Fortunately, the ability to detect small changes in iron nutrition in the population has been greatly improved in recent years by better employment of a battery of iron status measurements, such as transferrin saturation, red cell protoporphyrin, and serum ferritin.[5] Moreover, better ways of using the information obtained are being developed, not only to assess anemia or iron deficiency but to measure the changes in the iron-replete population as well.[6,7] However, these laboratory investigations must be carefully performed and adequately standardized to ensure reliable results.[8]

Field trials are expensive and require several years to design, conduct, and analyze. In countries where the costs of preliminary field trials are prohibitive or where the high prevalence of iron deficiency anemia dictates immediate action, it would seem reasonable to forego a field trial and proceed directly to a National Fortification Program. In this case, the efficacy of fortification must be assessed by monitoring iron status in the population before and after implementation of the program. However, there are many factors that may contribute to changes in iron status in a given country so that evaluation of a nutritional intervention where there is no predictable effect (such as would be available with the information obtained from a field trial and the studies leading to it) may hamper the effort to gauge the effect of the policy per se. No single fortification strategy is suitable for worldwide use. In this chapter, we present the strategies for combatting iron deficiency that have been applied over the past decade in Chile. We present the studies done in fortifying infant milk formulas, infant weaning cereals, and hemoglobin-fortified cookies for preschool and school age children. Finally, we address iron supplementation in newborn infants and premature infants.

A. GENERAL SETTING

1. Characteristics of the Country

In order to set the scene for the fortification trials to be described, it becomes necessary to give some information about Chile, its population, economy, and health care delivery.

2. Population, Economy, and Health

The population of Chile was estimated to be 11.9 million in 1984. The annual growth rate is 1.7% based on a 1983 crude birth rate of 23 per 1000; fertility rate is 3.0 and the crude death rate is 6.1 per 1000. A continuing growth rate of 1.7% means that the population will double every 45 to 50 years. Chile is one of the most urbanized nations in Latin America, with the vast majority (83%) of the population residing in urban areas. Santiago, its capital, accounts for more than one third of the national population. Primary education is free, universal, and compulsory from the ages of 6 to 15 years, accounting for Chile's high literacy rate of 95%.

Although Chile depends largely on imports for much of its food and energy, it is considered one of the world's 35 middle-income countries and one of the most highly industrialized countries of Latin America. Generally, there is a close correlation between economic development and nutritional status of the infant population. In Chile, however, these long-term economic difficulties and dramatically increasing unemployment rates (from 6% in 1966 to 21% in 1984) did not result in the normally expected upward trend in malnutrition and infant mortality through 1982. This can be largely attributed to long standing government-sponsored intervention programs.

Generally mortality (6.1/1000) and life-expectancy indicators rank Chile high worldwide. Life expectancy at birth for both sexes is 67.0 years. In 1940, Chile had one of the highest infant (birth to 1 year) mortality rates of Latin America, 193/1000. Through the 1940s the rate steadily declined and by 1950 it was 136/1000 reaching 120 by 1960. This decline continued through the 60s and 70s and by 1983 the rate fell to 21.5/1000 live births standing today (1986) at 18.7‰. The dramatic improvement in infant mortality rate may be attributed to the decline in malnutrition and the significant reduction of respiratory and diarrheal illnesses which claimed thousands during the first year of life. The intensive program of supplemental nutrition aimed precisely at this age group has undoubtedly been a contribution as detailed later. Another factor contributing to the general improvement in health of infants is the increased percentage of hospital births. In 1983, 95% of all births occurred in hospitals, providing newborns early health assessment and treatment, including immunizations.

Recognizing the importance of child development and maternal health to infant well-being, the government formulated a legislative policy mandating maternal and child health programs. Such expanded health policies provided women with increased access to pre- and postnatal care. Records of weight gain, blood pressure, health, and nutrition status are maintained in all who are enrolled in these programs.

The National Health Services (NHS) was created in 1952 to integrate the independent systems serving different populations.

3. Food and Nutrition Profile

The improvement in child nutritional status is attributed to many factors: health and nutrition control programs, milk distribution programs, treatment programs for malnourished children, and increased in hospital-based births; improve a decrease in the percentage of low-birth-weight newborns, family planning programs, expanded social welfare programs, and improvements in sanitation.

The unacceptably high rates of anemia in Chile, however, prompted iron fortification studies and the development of recent nutrition intervention programs. Yet, recognizing that nutrition intervention programs directed at eradicating specific health problems are likely to be only palliative and short term unless accompanied by long-range efforts to significantly promote social, health, economic, and educational development, the authorities made its nutrition policy an integral part of the national socioeconomic development. A variety of delivery systems have been utilized including existing health and education facilities and others established expressly to provide specialized services to specific target groups. The following is a description of some of those programs directed at mothers and young children, population groups with the highest incidence of iron deficiency and the focus of the efforts to combat iron deficiency anemia detailed in this chapter.

4. National Supplementary Food Program (NSFP)

Administered by the Ministry of Health through primary health centers, the NSFP provides low-income children from birth to 5 years of age with full-fat (26% fat) powdered milk and weaning foods at no cost. Children of middle and upper income families do not participate in the program. Prior to 1983, infants (0 to 6 months) received 3 kg of powdered milk per month; those between 6 months and 2 years received 2 kg; those between 2 and 5 years received 1.5 kg of weaning foods containing 20% protein. Pregnant women were given 2 kg of powdered milk (12% fat) per month and lactating women 3 kg of powdered milk.

In 1980, 1,324,000 women and children received government-distributed milk. Over the course of the past 20 years, 12 to 30 million kg of powdered milk or milk substitutes have been distributed annually. The program reaches 86% of the children under 6 months of age, 91% of children between 6 months and 2 years, 79% from 2 to 6 years, and 70% of pregnant and lactating women. Long-term experience with this program has facilitated the study of iron deficiency and the introduction of fortification programs.

In conjunction with the milk distribution program, also administered by the Ministry of Health, is the monthly health care program. The program includes growth and development monitoring, nutrition education, encouragement of breast feeding, immunizations, psychosensory stimulation for those with delayed development, family planning, and prenatal care.

5. Targeted Food Distribution Program

In 1974, a targeted food distribution program was designed to provide additional foods to indigent families with one or more children with or at risk of malnutrition. The purpose of this program was to improve the nourishment of the entire family. Foods delivered through the primary care centers to participating families include milk, rice, wheat, and oils. The criteria for participating in the program were (1) low-birth-weight newborns; (2) infants with poor weight gain for 2 consecutive months; (3) mothers less than 20 years old; (4) families with more than 5 children; and (5) families with significant socioeconomic handicaps. The program received support from international agencies through 1983 and is now incorporated into the national budget under the risk categories previously described.

6. Nursery School Feeding Program

Experience has shown that free distribution of food to poor families is not sufficient to prevent malnutrition among preschool children. Moreover, the conditions of poverty are known to have other deleterious effects on physical and mental development. Recognizing this, the government of Chile operates nursery school garden centers for children under 6 years of age. Located primarily in poor neighborhoods, these centers address not only children's educational and social needs, but their nutritional needs as well. There are presently 500 centers in urban areas and 350 outside the cities serving 105,000 children. They provide a complete food program, meeting 100% of the children's nutritional requirements. This program has recently been integrated with the school lunch program operated by the Ministry of Education.

7. School Breakfast and Lunch Program

Another food supplementary program, with the objective of improving childhood nutrition, is the School Lunch and Breakfast Program. Although some form of food distribution through the school system dates as far back as 1921, the program as currently structured started in 1966.

More than 7000 schools throughout the country participate in this program. On the average 950,000 breakfasts (400 kcal) and 545,000 lunches (850 kcal) are provided on school days to children in participating schools. These meals represent 80% of the recommended allowance for calories during school days.

II. FIELD TRIALS OF FORTIFIED FOODS

A. INFANCY
1. Cow's Milk Formulas
a. Background

Infancy is a period of particularly high risk for the development of iron deficiency. Neonatal stores are exhausted at 4 to 6 months of age in the term infant, much earlier in the premature. After this age, the infant is dependent on the diet for sources of iron, a diet which is usually monotonous and low in bioavailable iron. Unless there is additional iron in medicinal form or as food fortification, no less than one third of infants will develop anemia by 9 to 18 months of life. Two thirds will have biochemical evidence of iron deficit. This is true also for breast-fed children. Fortified infant milk or cereal is not available in Chile nor is there a practical means of providing supplemental iron. Thus, the surveys conducted in Chile show that 28 to 31% of infants 6 to 24 months of age have anemia, while biochemical evidence of iron deficiency is present in 43 to 65%.[9] The present and possible long-term consequences are unforeseen, however, evidence is mounting that behavioral derangements exist[10,11] and may not be readily reversible.[12]

The sequential approach to infant food fortification in four milk studies is described, a soy-based formula trial for artifically fed infants and a rice cereal fortified with hemoglobin iron as a weaning food in breast-fed infants.

b. Milk Study 1

In Chile, a large percentage of infants receive milk distributed by the National Health Service free of cost (part of NSFP). During this study, the program gave 3 kg of milk per month from 1 to 6 months of age and 2 kg up to 2 years of age. Milk, the main caloric source for the infant, can be easily fortified during its processing. Previous studies have demonstrated that fortified formulas can be utilized in the prevention of iron deficiency.[13-15] With this background, in 1972 we decided to determine the feasibility of enriching the partially skim (12% fat) powdered milk given out at that time with iron. Skim milk was fortified with 15 mg of iron as ferrous sulfate per 100 g of powder. At this enrichment level, there were no organoleptic changes and the shelf-life studies demonstrated that it could be kept at ambient temperature in polyethylene bags for at least 1 year. Radioisotope studies showed a mean absorption of 3 to 4%.[16]

This fortified formula was tested in the field in three NHS clinics where 603 infants were selected with the requisite of being healthy term infants, spontaneously weaned before 3 months of age. These infants were randomly assigned to a group treated with fortified milk or to a control group, which received the same milk that had not been fortified. Both milk preparations were administered for 1 year beginning at 3 months of age. At 3, 9, and 15 months of age, the iron status of these infants was evaluated. A reduction in the percentage of anemic infants from 34.6% in the control group to 12% was found at 15 months of age in the subjects who received the fortified formula. When only the subjects who had consistently consumed the fortified formula according to the stool iron determinations (*vide infra*), anemia was present in 9.9% of infants at 15 months. Similar findings were reported at 9 months, with somewhat higher levels of anemia (Figure 3). Even though a significant reduction of anemia was achieved, these results were not considered optimal probably because of the low bioavailability of the iron added to the nonmodified milk and by intrafamilial dilution, i.e., the consumption of this product by other members of the family.[17]

c. Milk Study 2

To improve the outcome of this study it was necessary to

1. Increase the bioavailability of the iron in fortified formula. With the knowledge ac-

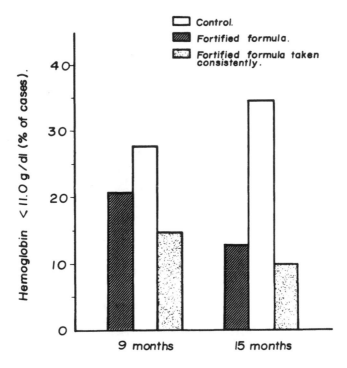

FIGURE 3. Prevalence of anemia at 9 and 15 months of age in infants
receiving nonfortified milk (control) or low-fat milk fortified with ferrous
sulphate (Milk Study 1). Infants taking milk consistently were defined
according to stool iron measurement. (From Stekel, A., et al., in *Nutrition
Intervention Strategies in National Development*, Underwood, B. A., Ed.,
Academic Press, New York, 1983, 317. With permission.)

quired in the interim of the enhancing effect in the absorption of iron produced by
ascorbic acid, the result of increasing concentrations of ascorbic acid was measured
in a double isotope absorption study.[18] It was appreciated that concentrations of ascorbic
acid equal to or above 100 mg/100 g of powdered milk significantly increased the
absorption of iron (Figure 4). In 1976, by the time these results were obtained, the
National Health Service had substituted the partially skim milk with a full-fat milk
with 26% fat. Thus, the decision was made to fortify this milk with 15 mg of iron as
ferrous sulfate and add 100 mg of ascorbic acid per 100 g of powder. In this case,
the geometric mean of iron absorption was brought up to 11%.[18] The enhancing effect
of ascorbic acid on iron absorption was shown to have a duration of at least 1 year
when this milk was vacuum-packed in tin cans.

2.   Discourage intrafamilial dilution. Milk was slightly acidified biologically by the utilization of *Streptococcus lactis*. Acidification has the purpose of discouraging the
consumption by other members of the family group, since it made the product un-
palatable for adults but perfectly acceptable to infants. This product was additionally
enriched with vitamins A and D (Table 2).

The effectiveness of this product was determined in a field trial performed in three NHS
clinics where 554 infants spontaneously weaned before 3 months of age with birth weights
about 2500 g were selected.[17] The infants were randomly assigned to the fortified or control
group. Both products were administered from 3 to 15 months of age in the quantities and
directions usually given by the NPSF. Solid foods were initiated similarly in both groups
with fruits at 3 months of age, a meat vegetable soup at 4 months of age, eggs and legumes
at 6 months, and at 9 to 12 months, the addition of table foods. Every 15 d, a field nurse

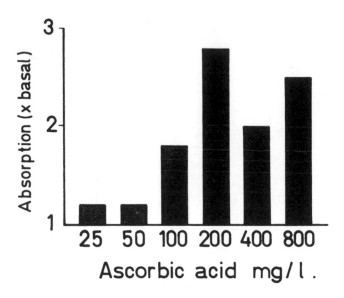

FIGURE 4..   Effect of ascorbic acid on the availability of fortification iron in milk. There were no significant differences when adding 100 mg/l or more. (From Stekel, A., et al., *Arch. Latinoam. Nutr.*, 33, 33, 1983. With permission.)

TABLE 2
Composition of an Acidified Milk
Formula Fortified with Iron and
Ascorbic Acid (per 100 g of powder)

Fat	26 g
Nonfat solids	68 g
Iron (as FeSO4)	15 mg
Ascorbic acid	100 mg
Vitamin A	1500 I.U.[a]
Vitamin D	400 I.U.[a]
Acidity	2.4 g lactic acid

[a]   I.U., International units.

performed a survey recording the food that was consumed by the family and the acceptability of the formula. Serial stool samples were obtained for the determination of iron in stools as an additional mean to monitor the consumption of this iron-fortified formula.[19] At 3, 9, and 15 months of age, a blood sample was taken for the following determinations: hematocrit, hemoglobin, serum iron, total iron-binding capacity, free erythrocyte protoporphyrin and serum ferritin in 198 infants at 9 months of age and 184 at 15 months. The acceptability field survey showed that the fortified milk was consistently consumed by at least 90% of all infants throughout the study. Initially, both groups presented identical iron nutrition. At 9 and 15 months of age, there were highly significant differences ($p < 0.001$) in favor of the iron fortified group in all the laboratory measures of iron nutrition (Figure 5). At 9 months of age, the frequency of anemia had been reduced from 34.7% in the control group to only 7.5% in the fortified group. The values at 15 months of age were 27.8 and 1.6%, respectively. We also appreciated at 9 and 15 months of age a significant reduction in the subjects with serum ferritin <10 μg/l in the fortified group, implying not only that anemia was erradicated, but that iron stores were actually improved (Figure 6). Acceptability was further evaluated by the stool iron measurements, where a clear-cut difference could be

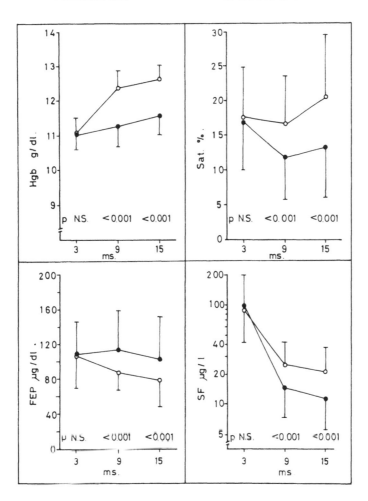

o———o Fortified milk   •———• Unfortified milk

FIGURE 5.   Pilot field study of Milk Study 1 showing mean and range of 1 SD of values for hemoglobin (Hgb), saturation of transferrin (Sat %), free erythrocyte protoporphyrin (FEP), and serum ferritin (SF) at 3, 9, and 15 months of age. (From Stekel, A., et al., in *Nutrition Intervention Strategies in National Development*, Underwood, B. A., Ed., Academic Press, New York, 1983, 317. With permission.)

observed between those infants in the non-fortified and the fortified group. From all those who were considered fortified milk consumers according to the surveys, only 89% complied as judged by the stool iron level. This demonstrates that a survey, even if performed at frequent periodic intervals by trained personnel can be as much as 10% in error. Moreover, great differences were evident in iron status between infants in the fortified group that were consumers and those who were nonconsumers (Figure 7).[19] This field study demonstrated that the acidified-fortified formula with added ascorbic acid improved iron nutrition significantly in these infants and was capable of practically eradicating the presence of anemia.[20]

d. Milk Study 3

The following step was to study the effect of this milk under the conditions of normal distribution in the National Health Service Clinics.[21] With this purpose, two cohorts of infants were chosen from all the clinics of the central area of Santiago, of whom a subset

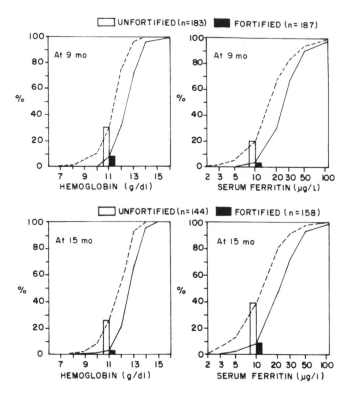

FIGURE 6.   Cumulative frequency distribution for hemoglobin and serum ferritin at 9 and 15 months of age of infants in Milk Study 2.

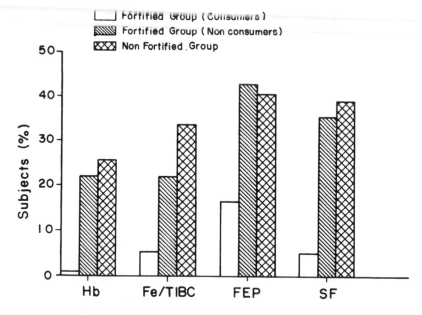

FIGURE 7.   Percent of subjects in Milk Study 2 with abnormal values for hemoglobin (Hb <11 g/dl), saturation of transferrin (Fe/TIBC <9%), free erythrocyte protoporphyrin (FEP >100 µg/dl RBC), and serum ferritin (SF <10 ng/ml). The fortified group was separated into consumers and nonconsumers based on stool iron determination. (From Pizarro, F., et al., *Am. J. Clin. Nutr.*, 45, 484, 1987. With permission.)

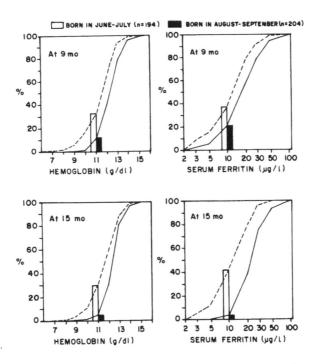

FIGURE 8. Cumulative distribution plots in Milk Study 3 for hemoglobin and serum ferritin at 9 and 15 months for infants given nonfortified milk (born in June to July) and those provided fortified, acidified formula (born in August to September).

of 1239 were followed longitudinally. Those infants born in June and July 1978 received the unfortified full-fat milk distributed normally by the NPSF and those born on the 2 following months (August and September) were offered the acidified-fortified milk throughout the study. If the infants were thought not to tolerate the formula, regular milk could be obtained by the parent on request. The cohorts were not different in birth weight, socioeconomic level, maternal age, or parity. The length of breast feeding was also similar in both groups, suggesting that the introduction of the formula, whether it was fortified or not, did not influence the duration of breast feeding in this setting where lactation is actively encouraged.

The acceptability of the fortified-acidified milk varied between 70 to 80% under these conditions, slightly lower than the 90% observed in the more tightly controlled pilot field trial. However, it was hard to determine if the reported lack of acceptability was really infant intolerance or the desire of the parent to obtain the regular milk which could be used by the whole family. In a further subset of approximately 200 infants per group, the iron nutritional status was determined. At 9 and 15 months of age, significant differences were noted between both groups in all the measures of iron nutrition. Anemia was present at 9 months in 11.8% of the fortified infants vs. 32.5% in the non-fortified infants. At 15 months, the values were of 5.5 and 29.9%, respectively (Figure 8). Further analysis of the effects of the duration of the administration of fortified food, showed that at 15 months of age, 3.8% of those infants that received formula for 10 months or more presented the anemia compared to 12.5% of those infants who received fortified milk for less than 10 months. In this large regional field study, we demonstrated that under the usual conditions of milk distribution by the NSFP, this fortified product was fairly well accepted and remained significantly effective in reducing the prevalence of iron deficiency.

e. Milk Study 4

The implementation of a National Program of Fortification on the basis of the acidified-

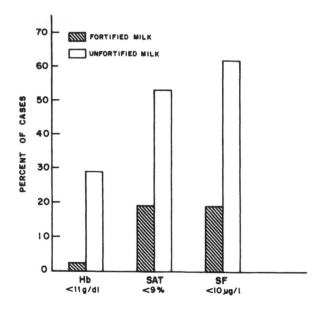

FIGURE 9. Percent of infants in Milk Study 4 with abnormal values for hemoglobin (Hb), saturation of transferrin (Sat), and serum ferritin (SF).

fortified milk presented, however, some inconveniences. This formula had an additional cost of 10 to 15% due mainly to the processing that was required for acidification and for the vacuum-sealed tin cans. Additionally, not all the providers of milk to the NSFP were equipped to manufacture this acidified product. It was also recognized that uncertainty existed whether the acidified milk would be equally popular and well accepted by the consumers, since this product could not be used for other members of the family. In view of these facts, the decision was made to test this same product but omitting acidification.

The radioisotope absorption studies showed that the iron bioavailability of the nonacidified formula was similar to that of the acidified product. In a pilot field study, identical in design to Milk Study 2, 190 infants were studied for the effect of this nonacidified formula given from 3 to 12 months of age. The acceptability of this product was again excellent. At 9 and 12 months of age, the iron status of infants showed highly significant differences ($p < 0.001$) in favor of the fortified group in all the laboratory measures evaluated. At the end of study, 12 months of age, the fortified group showed virtual absence of anemia, whereas 29.1% of the nonfortified group infants were anemic (Figure 9). Important changes were also appreciated in the percentage of deficiency according to other iron measures. We concluded that this nonacidified, fortified milk was as effective as the acidified milk in the prevention of iron deficiency with the advantages of a lower additional cost, less implementation needed for its elaboration, and dismissal of consumer acceptability doubts.

f. Therapeutic Trial

At the age of 12 months, when infants ended the field trial in study 4, they received a therapeutic trial of oral ferrous sulfate at 3 to 4 mg Fe^{2+} per kilogram per day for 3 months that was monitored by weekly visits and measurements of the amount of medication remaining. Only those receiving a total of 1250 mg of Fe were included in the analysis at 15 months. In the fortified group, 41 complied with this requirement, 71 in the nonfortified group. Not surprisingly, there were highly different hematologic values after the iron supplementation in the 71 unfortified infants. In the fortified group, mean hemoglobins were not statistically different before and after therapy; however, highly significant differences

TABLE 3
Effect of a Therapeutic Trial of Oral Iron between 12 and 15 Months of Age on Iron Status of Infants in a Fortification Trial

	Age	Hgb g/dl	MCV fl	Fe/IBC %	FEP µg/dl	SF[a] ng/ml
Nonfortified milk n = 71	12 m	11.2 ± 1.4	67 ± 7	9.1 ± 5.3	154 ± 86	8(4—17)
	p	0.0001	0.0001	0.0001	0.0001	0.0001
	15 m	12.4 ± 1.0	72 ± 4	15.3 ± 6.8	93 ± 31	17(9—32)
Fortified milk n = 41	12 m	12.6 ± 1.0	71 ± 6	15.4 ± 6.9	93 ± 38	18(10—32)
	p	NS	0.005	NS	0.001	0.05
	15 m	12.7 ± 0.7	75 ± 4	18.2 ± 7.9	75 ± 23	22(12—41)

Note: Mean ± SD.

[a] Geometric mean and range of 1 SD.

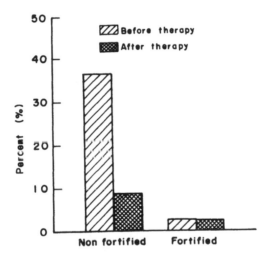

FIGURE 10.   Prevalence of anemia (Hb <11 g/dl) before and after therapeutic iron trial in the nonfortified and fortified infants of Milk Study 4.

were observed in MCV, FEP, and SF. (Table 3). We further compared the differences in the prevalence of anemia at 12 months using two criteria: (1) the level of hemoglobin (<11 g/dl) and (2) the response to the therapeutic trial of iron (increase of >1 g/dl of Hgb). Those infants receiving fortified milk had anemia by the Hgb criterion in 2% of the cases, whereas when the response criterion was used the prevalence of anemia increased to 12%. In the nonfortified group, the rise was also significant (from 36 to 48%) (Figure 10). However, the percentage of anemic infants after the trial was identical in the fortified group, whereas in the nonfortified infants the percent decreased from 34% to only 8% (Figure 11). The improvement in iron deposits expressed as the drop in the percentage of infants with SF <10 ng/ml is significant in the fortified group (from 10 to 5%) and dramatic in the nonfortified infants (58 to 13%) (Figure 12).

The therapeutic trial illustrates the fact that despite the use of multiple "state of the art" biochemical measures of iron status, a precise appreciation cannot be obtained from

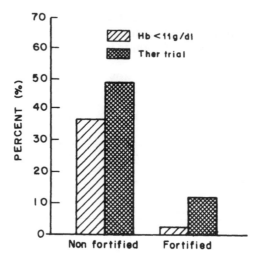

FIGURE 11.   Prevalence of anemia. Different criteria to measure anemia were used. A hemoglobin <11.0 g/dl before the therapeutic trial vs. the response of >1.0 g/dl in Hgb irrespective of level before the trial.

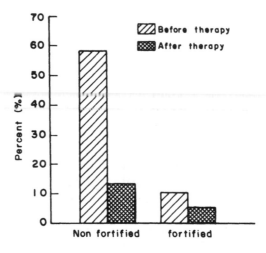

FIGURE 12.   Prevalence of iron depletion (serum ferritin <10 ng/ml) before and after the iron therapeutic trial in the nonfortified and fortified group of Milk Study 4.

the result of a fortification field trial, particularly to define the improvement in iron status in those with relatively good iron nutrition. Cook et al.[7] have designed methods to better assess the iron status of populations without the need of a therapeutic trial, however, these schemes have not been validated in infants and children.

2. Soy-Based Formulas
a. Background

Soy-based formulas are being increasingly utilized in infant feeding in many areas of the world. Recently, it was estimated that 10 to 15% of all formula-fed infants in the U.S. are receiving a soy-based formula.[22] Several reports indicate that soy products inhibit the

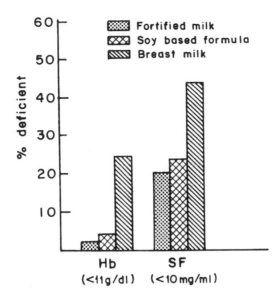

FIGURE 13. Percent of abnormal values for hemoglobin (Hb) and serum ferritin (SF) at 9 months of age in infants receiving (as only milk source): iron fortified cow's milk formula, soy-based fortified formula, or exclusive breast milk.

absorption of non-heme food iron and fortification iron.[23,24] On the other hand, it is reasonably presumed that the large amounts of iron commonly added to soy formulas would offset the inhibitory effects of soy. We studied the bioavailability of iron from a soy-based powdered formula (Prosobee® Mead-Johnson, Canada) and the effect of this preparation on the iron status of infants.[25] Iron absorption from this formula (iron added as ferrous sulfate, 12 mg/l; ascorbic acid, 54 mg/l) in 15 adult females was only 1.7%.

b. Field Trial of Soy Formula

The effect of this formula on iron nutrition was evaluated in a field trial in infants weaned spontaneously before 2 months of age and who received the formula *ad libitum* until 9 months of age. As controls, 45 infants were selected to receive a cow's milk formula fortified with ferrous sulfate (Fe, 15 mg/l; ascorbic acid, 100 mg/l) shown to be effective in preventing iron deficiency (Milk Study 4) and 49 additional exclusively breast-fed infants were also followed as controls. All subjects received solid foods (vegetables and meat) starting at age 4 months. Iron nutrition was determined only at 9 months. Infants fed soy formula, and iron-fortified cow's milk had similar mean values of hemoglobin, mean corpuscular volume, transferrin saturation, free erythrocyte protoporphyrin, and serum ferritin. Both formula groups differed significantly ($p < 0.05$) from the breast-fed group in all measures except free erythocyte protoporphyrin. Anemia (Hgb <11 g/dl) was present in only 4.3 and 2.2% of infants receiving the soy and the fortified formulas respectively vs. 27.3% in the breast-fed group. Differences in serum ferritin, were also common favoring the soy and fortified milk groups (Figure 13). The soy formula was prepared to contain 12 mg of iron and 1040 kcal/l. At the calculated iron absorption of 1.7%, the bioavailable nutrient density iron was 0.2 mg/1000 kcal. The average consumption of these infants was 750 kcal or 750 ml/d, thus the estimated absorbed iron would amount to 0.15 mg/d, a quantity insufficient to cover requirements. A weekly home visit for the completion of a dietary survey and acceptability measurement determined that sources of iron other than milk were negligible in all groups.

We found that despite the low iron bioavailability from this soy-based formula when measured in the adult, corroborating previous studies, infants fed with this formula as an exclusive source of milk up to 9 months of age, presented an unexpectedly good iron nutritional status.

This field trial illustrates contradictory results. In this case, the absorption study performed prior to the field test predicted low iron bioavailability and presumed insufficient iron nutriture. However, results still without clear explanations, showed excellent iron status, comparable to infants fed adequately tested iron fortified formulas.

3. Breast Feeding and Use of Weaning Cereals
a. Rationale

The duration and adequacy of breast feeding depends on a number of physiologic, nutritional, social, and cultural factors. The industrial revolution, urbanization, and the availability of alternate sources of infant milk have been implicated as causes for the decline in breast feeding all over the world. In the last few decades, Chile has been characterized by the existence of extensive programs of supplementary food distribution; however, the decline of breast feeding in Chilean mothers has not been temporally related to these programs of milk distribution. Apparently, the cause for the decline in breast feeding can be attributed to the fact that Chile began its urbanization early in the century, before industrialization became significant. Thus, the decline in breast feeding occurred before the onset of the National Supplementary Milk Distribution Program and has remained low, unaffected by its presence. The proportion of children from urban low class exclusively breast-fed at 3 months of age is similar in various studies performed between 1942 and 1977. The incidence ranges from 27 to 52%, most figures lying between 30 to 42%.[26]

When breast milk becomes insufficient to sustain normal growth, the common practice would be to introduce cow's milk supplements in a bottle, resulting in the rapid termination of breast feeding. In areas of the world where prolonged breast-feeding is prevalent, cereals represent a good mean of providing the necessary supplementary iron starting at about 4 to 6 months of age. Cereals, fed with a spoon as a gruel do not compete with suckling from the breast, thus contributing to the maintenance of successful breast feeding. Concurrently, it has become well recognized that between 4 and 6 months of age, caloric supplements must also be introduced in breast-fed infants as spoon-fed solids in such a way that breast feeding is not interfered with. Ideally, these solids should have a high caloric density and adequate protein quality. Additionally, they should provide the iron needed by breast-fed infants after about 4 to 6 months of age as it has been shown that even though the iron in breast milk is well absorbed, it will not confer adequate protection from iron deficit after that age.[15] Our laboratory[40] designed an extruded rice flour cereal fortified with 5% bovine hemoglobin concentrate that was prepared in an attempt to fill these requirements (Table 4). This cereal provides a suitable gruel preparation at 20% dilution and has an improved protein quality. It provides 14 mg of hemoglobin iron per 100 g with an estimated 0.6 mg of bioavailable iron. It is designed to be started at 4 months of age and to be increased gradually to 40 g/d by 6 months of age, thereby providing 140 kcal, and 0.84 mg of bioavailable iron. In the following field trial we have studied the influence of providing this cereal on the duration and adequacy of breast feeding as well as in the iron nutriture of infants attending a NHS clinic in Santiago.

b. Field Trial of Infant Cereal

Term infants (N = 255) who were being breast fed at 3 months of age were admitted to the study. One group of 123 randomly assigned infants received 1.5 kg of the cereal per month beginning at 4 months of age. The other group received the routine recommendations of the NHS, i.e., introduction of fruits at 3 months; vegetable-meat soup at 4 months of

145

TABLE 4
Characteristics of Infant Cereal Fortified with Bovine Hemoglobin

Extruded rice flour	95%
Bovine hemoglobin concentrate	5%
100 g of cereal provide:	
Kcal	360
Protein (g)	11.6
Fat (g)	0.3
Iron (mg)	14.0
Bioavailable iron per 100 kcal (mg)	0.6
Amino acid score (%)	60
PER[a] rice + Hgb	1.68
PER milk + rice + Hgb	3.05
PER casein control	2.91

[a] Shelf life in polyethylene bag, 2 years at room temperature. PER, protein efficiency ratio.

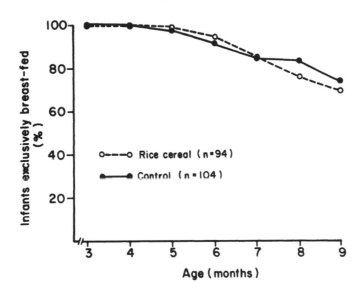

FIGURE 14. Breast feeding in two groups of infants after enrollment in a special promotion program beginning at 3 months of age. One group of infants received a rice cereal designed to supplement breast milk. (From Stekel, A., et al., in *Malnutrition: Determinants and Consequences*, Alan R. Liss, New York, 1984, 143. With permission.)

age; eggs, cereals, and legumes at 6 to 7 months; and regular table food at 9 to 12 months. The groups receiving the rice-hemoglobin cereal would introduce this cereal instead of the meat-vegetable soup either alone or mixed with small quantities of fruits or vegetables. All mothers were provided with powdered milk through the NSFP. The pediatric care was delivered by a team of physicians from INTA and field nurses performed house visits on a weekly basis for evaluation of morbidity and dietary patterns of the infants. The follow-up to 12 months of age was completed for 88 infants in the fortified group and 108 infants in the control group. Attrition was due mainly to migration. Acceptability of the cereal was good with 80% of the infants consuming more than half of the cereal prescribed daily up to 12 months of age.

The duration of exclusive breast feeding was similar in both groups (Figure 14). At 6

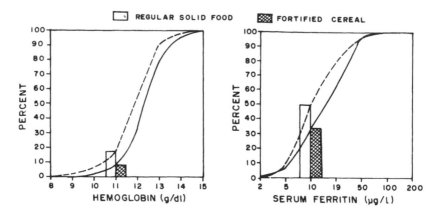

FIGURE 15.   Cumulative distribution plot of hemoglobin and serum ferritin of breast-fed infants at 12 months of age. One group received a rice cereal fortified with hemoglobin iron and the other regular meat-vegetable soups after 4 months of age.

months of age, 92% of all infants in the cereal group and 94% of those in the control group were still consuming breast milk as the only source of milk. Figures at 9 months were 73% and 69%, respectively. The high prevalence of prolonged breast feeding in this study can be attributed to the fact that this was a group of healthy term infants who were preselected as being exclusively breast fed at 3 months of age and subsequently breast feeding was strongly promoted by the physicians in the clinic and the nurses performing the home visits. It must be stressed that these figures were obtained during an active program of supplementary food distribution in which mothers are given cow's milk to take home. These data emphasizes the fact that the sole provision of free cow's milk to infants is not necessarily detrimental to the duration of breast feeding if it is accompanied by a program of breast feeding education and promotion by the Health Clinic Team.

At 12 months of age, there was a significant improvement of iron status in the supplemented group (Figure 15). The cumulative percentages depict the fact that anemia was present in 8% of fortified as opposed to 19% in the unfortified infants at 12 months of age. The percentage of anemia was higher in this study than in the fortified group in the trial of fortified acidified milk (Milk Study 2) where it was present in only 1.6% of infants at 12 months of age. The incidence of anemia in the control group was also lower (19 vs. 35%), demonstrating the partial protection from iron deficiency conferred by breast milk. Similar analysis applies to the proportion of low serum ferritin values. Fortified milk should be more efficient in eradicating iron deficiency since it is ingested in rather constant, measurable amounts and in our trials begun at 3 months of age, whereas this cereal is introduced at 4 months, reaching the amount designed to provide complete iron requirements only at 6 months of age. Also, the absolute amount ingested varied widely between and within infants. The growth of the infants in both groups was similar. Thus, we show that under the conditions of a controlled field trial, an infant weaning cereal significantly decreases iron deficiency in breast-fed infants without affecting duration of lactation. A major impact on prolonging breast feeding is accomplished by an active program of education and promotion of this practice by health personnel.

B.   School-Age Children
1.   Cookies Fortified with Bovine Hemoglobin
a. Background

The government sponsors two programs that address the nutritional needs of school children, the Nursery School Feeding Program and the School Breakfast Lunch Program. These national programs reach a significant proportion of the nutritionally vulnerable population, and have enjoyed long-standing support. On any given day, 90% of the eligible school children participate. For many years, three to four cookies (10 g each) have been given with milk or milk substitutes to participating children. Since cookies are a daily component of the children's diet, it seemed an ideal food vehicle to fortify with iron. Previous studies with ferrous sulfate and other inorganic iron substances proved unsatisfactory in cookies because of undesirable color or taste at levels of fortification used. Until the present investigations by INTA, there had been little experience using hemoglobin iron as a fortificant in cookies.

The purpose of the present investigation was to determine the absorbability, stability, efficacy, and acceptability of hemoglobin iron as a fortificant. Both the amount of iron in foods and its bioavailability vary considerably. Studies have demonstrated that iron enters into two common pools, the so-called heme iron and the non-heme iron pool. These pools have different absorption mechanisms. Heme iron, present in animal tissue, is well absorbed and its absorption relatively unaffected by diet composition. Callender et al.[27] and Turnbull et al.[28] demonstrated that hemoglobin iron is absorbed more efficiently than similar amounts of inorganic (non-heme) iron. Factors affecting non-heme iron absorption do not affect the bioavailability of heme iron. Unlike inorganic iron, heme iron is soluble in an alkaline medium which makes the intestinal pH more favorable for its absorption. Heme iron does not appear to be greatly affected by cooking.[29] Non-heme iron is principally present in cereals, vegetables, and fruits. Furthermore, there are some important animal sources of protein iron in infant nutrition that are poorly absorbed, e.g., iron in milk and eggs.

Because the diet of Chilean children is often chiefly made up of cereals and vegetables, it was considered that adding some non-heme iron to their diets would be unlikely to be significantly effective, especially when limited to the amounts that could be satisfactorily incorporated into a cookie. An equivalent amount of hemoglobin iron, it was hypothesized, would be significantly more effective. The use of hemoglobin as a food fortificant was suggested by Reizenstein in 1975.[30] This recommendation was based primarily on the characteristics of hemoglobin iron, and the relative poor absorption of non-heme iron fortificants.

Hemoglobin from animal blood is a relatively abundant source of iron and can be obtained through simple, low-cost technology. In addition to the isolation of hemoglobin from blood, the process permits the isolation of other blood proteins. These blood proteins can be used as protein supplements to the animal food. The key concern is to collect and process the blood in a sterile environment. Once dried, collected blood material is relatively safe for use.

In 1977, Hertrampf and co-workers[31] initiated investigations oriented to the possible use of hemoglobin in food fortification in Chile. Initially the studies were focused on the fortification of milk. Three heme iron concentrates were obtained from bovine red cells: hemoglobin with stroma, hemoglobin without stroma, and hemin. The three concentrates were tested separately. When added to milk in a concentration of 15 mg elemental iron per liter, there was no change in flavor and the color of the fortified milk was that of cafe-au-lait. Radioisotope absorption studies with intrinsic labeled hemoglobin preparations obtained from a Fe-labeled calf were conducted enrolling 70 infants 6 to 18 months of age. Absorption of each of the three heme iron concentrates was similar, with a geometric mean of 18.8%. Absorption of hemin was significantly higher in milk than in water, indicating that milk probably protected hemin from forming insoluble macromolecular aggregates. Hemoglobin added to milk, however, produced rapid rancidity of the product due to the oxidation of fat in the powdered milk. Hemoglobin fortification of milk was thus judged to be impractical. The lower fat content of cookies prompted studies of their use in heme fortification. During 1980 to 1982, INTA conducted studies to explore the feasibility of fortifying cookies with heme and, subsequently, the practicability of incorporating the cookies into the national program directed at school children.[32]

TABLE 5
Proximate Composition and Iron Content of
the Control and 6% BHC-Fortified Cookies

	Control	6% Fortification
Moisture (%)	6.4	4.6
Protein (N × 6.25) (%)	8.4	13.5
Ether extract (%)	11.0	11.0
Ash (%)	1.0	1.1
Nitrogen-free extract (%)	73.3	69.8
Iron (mg/100 g)	2.3	19.6

From Asenjo, J. A., et al., *J. Food Sci.*, 50, 795, 1985. With permission.

In order to prepare the Bovine Hemoglobin Concentrate (BHC), at the time of slaughter, whole blood was collected with sodium citrate as the anticoagulant. The blood was maintained at 4°C and within 3 to 6 h was separated into plasma and red cell fractions in a laboratory refrigerated centrifuge. The plasma was collected separately for use as protein for supplement. The red cells were washed three times with 0.9% sodium chloride and freeze dried at 26 to 30°C and at 0.1-mmHg chamber pressure. Microbial testing was conducted on all batches to ensure compliance with standards.

b. Pilot Fortification of Cookies

Cookies were fortified with 4, 6, or 8% BHC. The basic ingredients were wheat flour, liquid sugar, and hydrogenated lard. Monocalcium phosphate, sodium bicarbonate, and vanilla extract were used as additives. In addition, to avoid rancidity, an equal mixture of antioxidants, butylhydroxyanisol and butylhydroxytoluene were used. Cookies used in the school breakfast/lunch program contained the same ingredients as the fortified cookies with the exception of the BHC. The cookies were manufactured in a local factory in accordance with standard practice, consisting of: (1) dry-mixing of flour, BHC, additives, and antioxidants; (2) addition of hydrogenated lard and liquid sugar and kneading the mixture to a homogenous consistency; and (3) molding in an automatic machine and baking in a continuous horizontal electric oven for 10 min at 270°C.

Sensory evaluations of appearance, flavor, aroma, and texture were performed by a panel of ten judges and included two replications of each test. A seven point rating scale was used (7 = excellent; 1 = very poor). The order of presentation to the judges was randomized. In order to complement the quantitative information, the samples were described and the most relevant sensory characteristics noted. The judges detected no qualitative differences between the 4% and the 6% fortified cookies. The 8% cookies were rejected because of their poor appearance and flavor. In order to supply the highest possible amount of iron and protein, the cookies with 6% BHC were chosen as the most suitable for further study.

In comparison with the standard cookies regularly used in the breakfast program, the 6% fortified cookies had by proximate analysis, a lower moisture content, it was 1.6 times higher in protein content and 8 times higher in iron content (Table 5).

Amino acid analysis (Table 6) demonstrates that in comparison to the control cookies, the fortified cookie had a higher value for all essential amino acids except isoleucine. A significant difference between the fortified and unfortified cookies was that lysine was 73% deficient in the unfortified cookie and only 8% deficient in the fortified cookie. As a result, the amino acid score of the unfortified cookie was 28.6 and that of the fortified cookie 40.3, with isoleucine as the first limiting amino acid. Isoleucine is very abundant in cow's milk;

TABLE 6
Amino Acid Composition of the Control and Fortified Cookies
(6% BHC)

	g/100 g of Protein		
Amino acid	Control	Fortified	FAO/OMS pattern (1973)
Essential			
Lysine	1.46	5.01	5.44
Threonine	2.16	2.65	4.00
Methionine & cystine	1.21	1.49	3.52
Valine	3.86	6.45	4.96
Phenylalanine & tyrosine	6.45	7.49	6.08
Leucine	6.66	10.60	7.04
Isoleucine	3.03	1.61	4.00
Tryptophan	(a)	(a)	0.96
Nonessential			
Arginine	3.06	3.56	
Aspartic acid	4.40	7.90	
Serine	3.97	4.24	
Glutamic acid	41.69	28.16	
Proline	(b)	(b)	
Glycine	3.46	4.13	
Alanine	2.97	6.53	
Histidine	1.85	4.24	

[a] Tryptophan was not determined.
[b] Trace amounts.

From Asenjo, J. A., et al., *J. Food Sci.*, 50, 795, 1985. With permission.

therefore, when the fortified cookies are consumed simultaneously with cow's milk or a milk substitute, the amino acid score of the meal increases markedly.

The fortified cookie maintained good organoleptic characteristics for up to 7 months when kept at an ambient temperature (17 to 20°C) in oxygen- and light-proof packaging.

For the bioavailability studies, intrinsically labeled red cells were obtained by injecting a calf with ^{55}FeCl. The calf was slaughtered 2 months later and the radioactive BHC was prepared by freeze drying the red cells, as previously described. Labeled cookies (1 kg) were prepared using 60 g of a mixture of cold (nonradioactive) BHC to give an activity of 2.1 μCi ^{55}Fe/30 g of cookies. The cookies were prepared as previously described. The radioactivity in these cookies was extremely low and the dosage was approved by the Committee of Human Experimentation of the University of Chile.

Absorption studies were performed using 15 healthy children, 2 to 7 years of age. On day 1, subjects consumed 30 g of fortified cookies containing 5.5 mg of elemental iron and 2.1 μCi ^{55}Fe. On day 2, subjects were given 50 ml of an aqueous aolution of ferrous ascorbate containing 2 mg of elemental iron and 0.7 μCi ^{59}Fe as a reference dose. Absorption was determined on day 15 from the circulating radioactivity. Mean absorption of heme iron in cookies was 19.7%.

The following calculations can be made from the test results to estimate the amount of iron supplied by the fortified cookies. Each 30 g of cookies, the daily amount provided in the School Breakfast/Lunch program, contains 1.8 g BHC, or approximately 5 mg heme iron. With a mean absorption of 20%, the daily requirement of 1 mg absorbed iron will be supplied by the fortified cookies.

c. Pilot Field Study

A pilot field study with the 6% BHC-fortified cookies was conducted in two schools in the city of Santiago. The two schools were selected on the basis of their location in a low income area of the city, having adequate coverage by School Breakfast/Lunch Program, and the willingness of parents and teachers to participate in the study. The study lasted 2 school years (March to November 1980 and March to November 1981). Children in one school received three 10 g fortified cookies together with a glass of milk or milk substitutes (milk-wheat-soy drinks). Children in the other school continued receiving the standard three 10 g unfortified cookies with their milk. Cookies were given school days only (approximately 180 d/year) and eaten under the supervision of a teacher to ensure consumption. Once a week, a research nurse measured acceptance of the cookies by direct observation of their consumption. Children were required to leave the uneaten cookies in the dining area.

A random sample of 215 children (6 to 12 years) from each school was selected for hematological evaluation at the beginning of the study, at 7 months (end of the first school year), and at 15 months (end of the second year). A total of 169 children completed the study in the control group and 180 in the fortified group. Age, sex, socioeconomic background, and nutrition status as measured by anthropometry were similar in both groups. Acceptance and tolerance of the cookies was excellent. On the average, less than 2.5% of the served cookies were left uneaten throughout the 2 years of the study with no significant differences between the fortified and unfortified products.

Unfortunately, interpretation of hematological effects in this study is difficult because the two groups of children had good iron status at the beginning of the study. There were no initial differences between the groups in hemoglobin concentration, transferrin saturation, or serum ferritin. Hemoglobin values were uniformly high in both groups and no child had anemia (hemoglobin concentration below 12 g/dl). At the end of the trial, there was a small but statistically significant difference in hemoglobin concentration in favor of the fortified group. Anemia was present in 3.1% of the control group and 0.6% in the fortified group. When focusing on a subgroup with higher iron requirements, i.e., females over 10 years of age, however, differences became more apparent. Ferritin after 18 months of study was higher in the fortified (27.2 vs. 17.3 ng/ml, $p < 0.05$). No differences were immediately evident in hemoglobin. However, depicting Hgb in a cumulative plot, the fortified group shows no anemia with the control group having 6.2% of Hgb <12.5 g/dl. When the lower cutoff level for ferritin is set at 10 ng/ml, 10.9% of the girls in the control group were deficient vs. 6% in the fortified group. Low iron stores are better distinguished, however, when values below 20 ng/ml are considered. Then, 47% of control girls fall below 20 ng/ml vs. only 13.5% in the fortified group, a difference which is statistically significant (Figure 16). In conclusion, the fortification cookies were well accepted and tolerated by the school children. The hematological effects observed in these iron-replete children are not prominent because of the original good iron status of the subjects. Nevertheless, ferritin, an accepted indicator of iron stores, demonstrated a significant difference in favor of the fortified group.

d. National Program

At the end of 1980, before the field study was completed, it was decided to introduce the BHC-fortified cookies to the National School Breakfast/Lunch Program. Officials in charge of the program concluded, on the basis of the initial absorption studies, that there was sufficient scientific justification for using the cookie in the school program. These studies had demonstrated that the cookies would supply the required absorbable iron. Moreover, the protein quality of the fortified cookies was a marked improvement over the unfortified cookies.

Several steps were necessary in order to develop a national program: (1) definition and requisites of BHC for human consumption, (2) development of large scale production of BHC, (3) transfer of technology from small scale fortified cookie manufacture at the University to large scale industrial production, and (4) modification of contacts between JNAEB

151

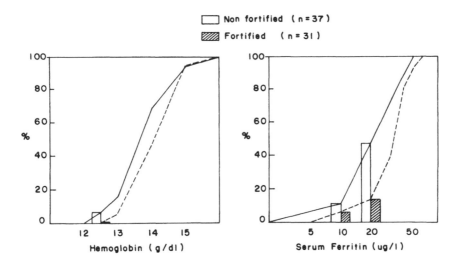

FIGURE 16. Cumulative distribution plot of hemoglobin and serum ferritin of girls older than 10 years at the end of the second year of the pilot field trial of hemoglobin fortified cookie.

and concessionaries in order to replace unfortified with fortified cookies and provide payment for additional costs involved.

A norm was prepared on the basis of the studies performed at INTA. This norm, entitled "Blood for Human Consumption — Dehydrated Concentrate of Corpuscular Fraction", defined BHC as a "fine powder of dark-red color obtained by centrifugation and further dehydration of the corpuscular fraction of blood of slaughtered animals". It specified the requisites of the product in terms of the quality of the raw materials, organoleptic characteristics, chemical and physiochemical characteristics, microbiological requisites, packaging, storing, and refrigeration.

Although there is an established market for bovine plasma, a product that is used in the meat industry, there was no market for red blood cells. The possibility of drying the red cells to produce BHC for the cookies fortification program made the project economically feasible. The drying plant was built in 1980. From a technical point of view, the main problem was expanding the drying conditions that had been used in the laboratory to an industrial level, and maintaining a suitable product that would comply with standards established by the norms. This was accomplished by close collaboration between INTA investigators and representatives of the new industry. In practice, most of the blood that is needed for the national program is obtained from the main slaughterhouse in Santiago. Processing entails initial collection of the blood in stainless steel containers, transfer of the product to fiberglass tanks, transport of the blood-filled tanks at ambient temperature to the drying plant, separation of plasma from the red blood cells, and spray drying the red blood cells in a Galaxie spray dryer at an entrance temperature of 160°C and exit temperature of 85°C. All blood is processed and dried within 4 h of collection.

Fortified cookies must conform to rigidly established norms. In addition to quality control procedures instituted by each manufacturer, random samples of fortified cookies from all the manufacturers are analyzed by INTA each month. Samples are subjected to microbiological analyses, physicochemical analyses (proximate analysis), and sensory evaluations.

In 1984, the number of school children receiving breakfast was 950,000. To measure the impact in iron nutriture of the National Program, the province of Linares was left unfortified. The evaluation has been planned after 4 to 5 years of the initiation of the program, to allow for sufficient effect on iron status and avoid the difficulties in interpretation occuring in the pilot trial. The results are not yet available.

III. IRON SUPPLEMENTATION

If fortified foods are not available, it becomes necessary to introduce medicinal iron preparations to comply with the iron requirements not provided by the diet.

A. ORAL IRON SUPPLEMENTATION

The benefit of iron compounds for oral use has been widely demonstrated.[33,34] The iron salt most extensively utilized is ferrous sulfate due to its effectiveness and low cost. However, there are other iron salts which are at least equally adequate.[35] The American Academy of Pediatrics[36] has recommended that supplementation should be initiated not later than 4 months of age in term infants and not later than 2 months of age in preterm infants and required during the whole first year of life. The recommended dose is 1 mg/kg/d for term infants and 2 mg/kg/d for preterm infants, but not to exceed 15 mg/day.

1. Field Trial in Premature Infants

In a study in which 130 preterm newborns were evaluated,[41] half of the infants were given 2.5 mg/kg/d of iron as ferrous sulfate drops from 3 to 12 months of age. The remaining 65 infants received powdered milk that was acidified and fortified with 15 mg of elemental iron as ferrous ascorbate and 100 mg of ascorbic acid per 100 mg of powder, (the formula of Milk Study 3). The oral intake of this fortified milk and the medicinal preparations were reinforced and monitored periodically at weekly house calls performed by a field nurse. At 6, 9, and 12 months of age, those premature infants receiving the medicinal preparation of iron had significantly lower levels of hemoglobin. The percentage of anemic subjects in this group was 23.9% at 12 months of age, compared to only 4.2% in the infants that were given the fortified formula. As in other studies performed in children, there were no symptoms of intolerance attributable to the use of oral iron in either form. The unsatisfactory results obtained with use of medicinal oral iron are ascribed to lack of compliance despite the weekly supervision by a field nurse and the recognized high motivation level of mothers of premature infants.

2. Parenteral Iron Supplementation

Absorption of iron added to food is complicated by interfering substances present in the food source. The use of medical preparations presents similar problems when given with meals and, in addition, presents inconveniences derived from lack of compliance and, to a lesser degree, the chance of gastrointestinal intolerance. These difficulties could be circumvented by the administration of parenteral iron. The dose administered at a single neonatal visit could theoretically cover the entire requirement of iron for the first year of life. This product seems to be particularly useful in infants that for various reasons would be unavailable to fortification programs or periodic clinical control. Based on this rationale, we administered i.m. 150 mg of iron dextran to 261 term normal infants within the first 3 d of life.[42] No adverse side effects of consideration were observed in the immediate postnatal period or subsequently. Nine infants were lost to follow-up after discharge at 3 d of life. At 3, 9, and 15 months of age, we evaluated the iron status of these infants compared to 407 infants that had not been supplemented nor received fortified foods. At all the ages studies, there were significant differences in favor of the treated group for all laboratory parameters measured (Figure 17). Anemia was present in 1.9% of the supplemented infants at 9 months of age and 2.6% at 15 months of age, while these figures for the control group were of 29.7 and 31.2%, respectively. Similar results have been reported by other authors ,[37,38] however, Barry and Reeve in 1977[39] communicated in a retrospective study that the use of parenteral iron in the newborn period could be associated with an increase in the incidence of severe bacterial infections. This observation has limited further efforts to study the effect of par-

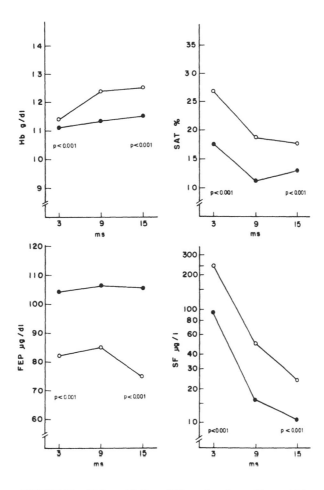

FIGURE 17. Values at 3, 9, and 15 months of age of hemoglobin (Hb), saturation of transferrin (Sat %), free erythrocyte protoporphyrin (FEP), and serum ferritin of infants who received intramuscular iron dextran (OO) and controls (●●).

enteral iron preparations in newborn infants until evidence is gathered that it would be of minimal risk. Before this issue is resolved, the use of parenteral iron should be considered as contraindicated in infants under the age of 3 months.

IN MEMORIAM

This chapter is dedicated to the memory of Abraham Stekel, M.D. (1940—1985), an internationally respected scientist, distinguished colleague, and dear friend. He gave generously of his time and talents to bring the benefits of hematologic and nutrition research to the children of Chile. A compassionate leader, he was a source of inspiration and encouragement. He leaves behind a legacy that will enrich the lives of those fortunate to have known and loved him, as well as the many he never knew but to whose well-being he devoted his life.

Born in Chile, Dr. Stekel received his medical degree from the University of Chile School of Medicine in Santiago. Following a short residency in his native country, he went to the U.S. to advance his education, studying under the guidance of Dr. Clement A. Finch at the University of Wisconsin and the University of Washington. After several years of intense work, he returned to Chile, committed to the investigation of iron deficiency and anemia. He was a pioneer in planning strategies to prevent this nutritional deficiency. His endeavors and successes have brought recognition to the Institute of Nutrition and Food Technology (INTA), a research institute of which he is a cofounder. In 1983, he was awarded the Swiss International Prize in Nutrition for his long-standing achievements.

Bold, taking risks when necessary, yet thoughtful and cautious in all decision-making, he did not confine himself to the ivory tower of this laboratory. He involved himself in reaching out to community and political leaders. He had a keen sense of social responsibility and strove to bring the results of his investigations to the disadvantaged, poorly nourished children of the world.

Chile has lost a great man of science. His death saddens us all. He will be sorely missed. He leaves behind a rich and enduring legacy.

REFERENCES

1. **Clydesdale, F. M. and Wiemer, K.,** Iron fortification of foods, in *Food Sciences and Technology. A Series of Monographs,* Academic Press, Orlando, FL, 1985.
2. **Acosta, A., Amar, M., Cornbluth-Szarfarc, S., Dillman, E., Fosi, M., Biachi, R. G., Grebe, G., Hertrampf, E., Kremenchusky, S., Layrisse, M., Martinez-Torres, C., Moron, C., Pizarro, F., Reynafarje, C., Stekel, A., Villavicencio, D., and Zuniga, H.,** The iron absorption from typical latinoamerican diet, *Am. J. Clin Nutr.,* 39, 953, 1984.
3. **Hallberg, L.,** Iron nutrition and food iron fortification, *Semin. Hematol.,* 19, 31, 1982.
4. **Hallberg, L.,** Bioavailable nutrient density: a new concept applied in the interpretation of food iron absorption data, *Am. J. Clin. Nutr.,* 34, 2242, 1981.
5. **Cook, J. D., Finch, C. A., and Smith, N. J.,** Evaluation of the iron status of a population. *Blood,* 48, 449, 1976.
6. **Cook, J. D. and Finch, C. A.,** Assessing iron status of a population, *Am. J. Clin. Nutr.,* 32, 2115, 1979.
7. **Cook, J. D., Skikne, B. S., Lynch, S. R., and Reusser, M. E.,** Estimates of iron sufficiency in the US population, *Blood,* 68, 726, 1986.
8. International Nutritional Anemia Consultative Group, Measurements of Iron Status. Nutrition: Washington Foundation, 1985.
9. **Rios, E., Olivares, M., Amar, M., Chadud, P., Pizarro, F., and Stekel, A.,** Evaluation of iron status and prevalence of iron deficiency in infants in Chile, in *Nutrition Intervention Strategies in National Development,* Underwood, B. A., Ed., Academic Press, New York, 1983, chap. 24.
10. **Lozoff, B. and Brittenham, G. M.,** Behavioral aspects of iron deficiency, in *Progress in Hematology,* Vol. 14, Brow, E., Ed., New York, 1985.
11. **Walter, T., Kovalsky, J., and Stekel, A.,** Effect of mild iron deficiency on infant mental development scores, *J. Pediatr.,* 102, 519, 1983.
12. **Deinard, A. S., List, A., Lindgren, B., Hunt, J. V., Chang, P. N.,** Cognitive deficits in iron-deficient and iron-deficient anemic children, *J. Pediatr.,* 108, 681, 1986.
13. **Marsh, A., Long, H., and Stierwalt, E.,** Comparative hematological response to iron fortification of a milk formula for infants, *Pediatrics,* 24, 404, 1959.
14. **Andelman, M. B. and Sered, B. R.,** Utilization of dietary iron by term infants, *Am. J. Dis. Child.,* 111, 45, 1966.
15. **Saarinen, U. M.,** Need for iron supplementation in infants on prolonged breast feeding, *J. Pediatr.,* 93, 177, 1978.
16. **Stekel, A., Olivares, M., Pizarro, F., Chadud, P., Lopez, I., and Amar, M.,** Absorption of fortification iron from milk formulas in infants, *Am. J. Clin. Nutr.,* 43, 917, 1986.
17. **Stekel, A., Olivares, M., Pizarro, F., Chadud, P., Cayazzo, M., López, I., and Amar, M.,** Prevention of iron deficiency in infants by milk fortification. I. A field trial with a low-fat milk, *Arch. Latinoam. Nutr.,* 36, 654, 1986.
18. **Stekel, A., Olivares, M., Pizarro, F., Amar, M., Chadud, P., Cayazzo, M., Llaguno, S., Vega, V., and Hertrampf, E.,** The role of ascorbic acid in the bioavailability of iron from infants foods, *Int. J. Vitam. Nutr.,* 55(Suppl. 27), 167, 1985.

19. **Pizarro, F., Amar, M., and Stekel, A.,** Determination of iron in stools as a method to monitor consumption of iron fortified products in infants, *Am. J. Clin. Nutr.,* 45, 484, 1987.
20. **Stekel, A., Olivares, M., Cayazzo, M., Chadud, P., Llaguno, S., and Pizarro, F.,** Prevention of iron deficiency by milk fortification. II. A field trial with a full fat milk, *Am. J. Clin. Nutr.,* 47, 265, 1988.
21. **Stekel, A., Pizarro, F., Olivares, M., Chadud, P., Llaguno, S., Cayazzo, M., Hertrampf, E., and Walter, T.,** Prevention of iron deficiency by milk fortification. III. Effectiveness under the usual operational conditions of a nation-wide food program, *Nutr. Int. Rep.,* 38, 1119, 1988.
22. Committee on Nutrition, Soy protein formulas. Recommendations for use in infant feeding, *Pediatrics,* 71, 359, 1983.
23. **Cook, J. D., Morck, T. A., and Lynch, S. R.,** The inhibitory effect of the soy products on non-heme iron absorption in man, *Am. J. Clin. Nutr.,* 34, 2622, 1981.
24. **Hallberg, L. and Rossander, L.,** Effect of a soy protein on non-heme iron absorption in man, *Am. J. Clin. Nutr.,* 36, 514, 1982.
25. **Hertrampf, E., Cayazzo, M., Pizarro, F., and Stekel, A.,** Bioavailability of iron in soy based formula and its effect on iron nutriture in infancy, *Pediatrics,* 78, 640, 1986.
26. **Mardones-Santander, F.,** History of breast feeding in Chile, *Food Nutr. Bull.,* 1, 15, 1979.
27. **Callender, S. T., Mallet, B. J., and Smith, M. D.,** Absorption of hemoglobin iron, *Br. J. Haematol.,* 3, 186, 1957.
28. **Turnbull, A., Cleton, F., and Finch, C. A.,** Iron absorption. IV. The absorption of hemoglobin iron, *J. Clin. Invest.,* 41, 1897, 1962.
29. **Reizenstein, P.,** Hemoglobin fortification of food and prevention of iron deficiency with heme iron, *Acta Med. Scand. Suppl.,* 1980.
30. **Reizenstein, P.,** Annotation. Cattle hemoglobin, a possible dietary iron supplement, *Br. J. Haematol.,* 31, 265, 1975.
31. **Hertrampf, E., Amar, M., and Stekel, A.,** Absorption of heme iron preparations given with milk in infants, presented at 12th Congr. Int. Soc. Hematology, Paris, 1978.
32. **Asenjo, J. A., Amar, A., Catagena, N., King, J., Hiche, E., and Stekel, A.,** Use of a bovine heme iron concentrate in the fortification of biscuits, *J. Food Sci.,* 50, 795, 1985.
33. **Mackay, H. M. M.,** Nutritional Anemia in Infancy with Special Reference to Iron Deficiency, His Majesty's Stationery Office, London, 1931.
34. **Sturgeon, P.,** Studies of iron requirements in infants and children. IV. Recommended daily dietary allowances, in *Iron in Clinical Medicine,* Wallerstein, R. O. and Mettier, S. R., Eds., University of California Press, Berkeley, 1958.
35. **Brise, H. and Hallberg, L.,** Absorbability of different iron compounds, *Acta Med. Scand.,* 171(Suppl. 376), 23, 1962.
36. Committee on Nutrition, Amercian Academy of Pediatrics, Iron supplementation for infants, *Pediatrics,* 58, 765, 1976.
37. **Tonkin, S.,** Maori infant health: trial of intramuscular iron to prevent anemia in maori babies, *N.Z. Med. J.,* 71, 129, 1970.
38. **Cantwell, R. J.,** Iron deficiency anemia of infancy: some clinical principles illustrated by the response of maori infants to neonatal parenteral iron administration, *Clin. Pediatr.,* 11, 443, 1972.
39. **Barry, D. M. J. and Reeve, A. W.,** Increased incidence of gram-negative neonatal sepsis with intramuscular iron administration, *Pediatrics,* 18, 353, 1965.
40. **Calvo, E.,** unpublished data.
41. **Rios, E.,** unpublished data.
42. **Olivares, M.,** unpublished data.

INDEX

developmental changes in, 46—50
    fall in, 35, 37
maternal-fetal relationships, 45—49
red cell mean corpuscular volume, 34, 37
serum ferritin in, 58—59

G

Gastric acid, diminished secretion of, 67
Gastrointestinal abnormalities, iron deficiency and, 67
Glossitis, 66, 69
Glutathione (GSH), 76—77, 79
Glutathione disulfide (GSSG), 76—77
Glutathione peroxidase (GSH-Px), 44, 76
Glutathione reductase (GR), 76—77
Glycan, 101
Glycoproteins, 2—4, 7
Glycosylation, 7
Golgi apparatus, 6
Growth needs, 44—45
Guinea pig milk, 95

H

Haber-Weiss reaction, 75
Hair, effects of iron deficiency on, 66
Half-life, 9
Haptoglobin-hemoglobin complex, 16, 20
Heart ferritin, 59—60
Heat sterilization, 121
Hematocrit values, 43
Hematopoiesis, 33—51, 60—62
    copper, interrelationship with, 41
    erythropoietin, role of, 41—42
    fetus, 34—35
    full-term infants, 45—51, see also Full-term infants
    growth needs, 44—45
    hemoglobin concentration, maintenance of, 35—39
    iron needs, 44—45, 47
    low-birth-weight infants, 34—36
    protein intake, 41—47
    selenium, role of, 39—40
    vitamin E, role of, 39—40
Hemoglobin, 10, 13—14
Hemoglobin concentration
    cord serum ferritin and, 46, 48
    full-term infants, 46—50
    low-birth-weight infants, 37—38
    human milk-fed very low-birth weight infants, 42—43
    maintenance of, 35—39
    racial difference, 47
    transferrin saturation, function of, 50
    yardstick for iron deficiency, 64
Hemoglobin synthesis, 15—16, 46, 57
Hemolysis, 44
Hemolytic anemia, 39, 80
Hemosiderin, 13—14
Hepatocytes, 6—7, 13, 16—17, 19, 90
Human lactoferrin, 101—102
Human milk, 87—107, see also Cow's milk

bioavailability of iron from, 88, 95—103, 110
ferritin, 90
forms of iron in, 88—91
iron absorption, 98
iron content of, 91—95
iron variation during lactation, 91—92
low molecular weight compounds, 90—91
maternal iron status, 92—94
protein-bound iron, 88—90
simulated, 101
xanthine oxidase, 89—91
Human milk-fed very low-birth-weight infants protein intake, role of, 41—47
Hyaline membrane disease, 78—79
Hydrogen peroxide, 75
Hydroxyl radical, 74—75
Hyperferemia, 18
Hyperoxia, 79—80
Hypoproteinemia, 41
Hypoxia, 79

I

Ice, craving for, 66, 69
Idiopathic hemochromatosis, 20, 59—60
Industrialized countries, iron deficiency, 128
Infancy, field trials of fortified foods, 134—136, see also Iron fortification
Infant cereals, 110—111, 117—118
    bioavailability of nonheme food iron, 113—114
    field trials of iron fortification of, 144—146
    iron content, 118
    iron fortification guidelines and regulation, 118
    iron preparations used to fortify, 119—121
Infant foods, see Baby foods
Infant formulas, 115—117
    casein predominant, 115
    heat sterilization, 121
    iron absorption, 98
    iron content, 117
    iron fortification guidelines and regulations, 115—117
    iron in, 109—126
    iron preparations used to fortify, 119
    milk-based, 115
    soy-based, 115
    whey predominant, 115
Infections, 97
Inflammations, 17, 20
Insulin, 41
Intracellular iron delivery, 9—12
Intrinsically labeled cow's milk, 98
Inverted gut sac system, 101
Iron, see also specific topics
    bioavailability in baby foods, 112—114
    forms in human milk, 88—91
    half-life, 9
    importance of, 2
    most important function, 64
    nature of, 2
    oxygen stress and, 81

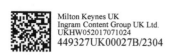

9 780367 450892